COLOUR GUIDE

D1592679

Forensic Medicine

John A.M. Gall BSc, MB, BS, PhD, MACLM, DMJ (Clin. & Path.)
Forensic Physician, Australian Forensic and Medico-Legal Consultants, and
Child Protection Unit, Monash Medical Centre, Melbourne, Australia
Formerly Forensic Physician, Victorian Institute of Forensic Medicine and
Honorary Senior Lecturer, Department of Forensic Medicine, Monash
University, Melbourne, Australia

Stephen C. Boos BS, MD
United States Air Force, Medical Corps
Air Force Medical Consultant in Child Abuse and Neglect, Armed Forces
Center for Child Protection
National Naval Medical Center, Bethesda, Maryland, USA

J. Jason Payne-James LLM, MB, BS, FRCS (Ed. & Eng.), DFM
Forensic Physician, Forensic Healthcare Services Ltd, London
Forensic Medical Examiner, Metropolitan Police Service and City of London
Police, London
Honorary Senior Research Fellow, Department of Gastroenterology and
Nutrition, Central Middlesex Hospital, London, UK

Elizabeth J. Culliford MB, BS (Hons Lond.), MRCP (UK), MACLM,
Grad. Dip. Forens. Med. (Monash)
Deputy Director, Government Medical Officer Services, South East Queensland
Region, Queensland Health, Queensland, Australia

CHURCHILL
LIVINGSTONE

EDINBURGH LONDON NEW YORK PHILADELPHIA ST LOUIS SYDNEY
TORONTO 2003

CHURCHILL LIVINGSTONE
An imprint of Elsevier Science Limited

Medical knowledge is constantly
changing. As new information
becomes available, changes in
treatment, procedures, equipment
and the use of drugs become
necessary. The authors and the
publishers have taken care to
ensure that the information given
in this text is accurate and up to
date. However, readers are
strongly advised to confirm that
the information, especially with
regard to drug usage, complies
with the latest legislation and
standards of practice.

First published 2003

ISBN 0-443-06499-7

British Library Cataloguing in Publication Data
A catalogue record for this book is available from
the British Library

Library of Congress Cataloging in Publication Data
A catalog record for this book is available from
the Library of Congress

The
publisher's
policy is to use
**paper manufactured
from sustainable forests**

Printed in China by RDC Group Limited

Commissioning Editor: Timothy
Horne
Project Development Manager:
Siân Jarman
Project Manager: Frances Affleck
Designer: George Ajayi

Preface

This volume in the Colour Guide series provides a concise overview of key areas in clinical forensic medicine amenable to photographic illustration. The text is not intended as a comprehensive coverage of the field but as a guide to the most important principles of clinical forensic medicine and an *aide mémoire* to common pitfalls. Practical advice is also given on the conduct of various forensic examinations, the collection of forensic specimens and documentation of findings; this will be of use to any healthcare practitioner who may become involved in medicolegal assessment or investigation for the judiciary, police or other body. In particular it will have relevance to postgraduate doctors at junior and senior grades, including forensic physicians, paediatricians (in hospital and community), other primary care physicians and general practitioners, accident and emergency specialists, specialists in genitourinary medicine and obstetrics and gynaecology who may be called upon to provide or interpret clinical forensic examinations. It will also be of considerable value to undergraduate medical and dental students and members of the legal profession.

Melbourne   J.A.M.G.
2003   S.B.
                                                             J.J.P.-J.
                                                             E.C.

Acknowledgements

The following are gratefully acknowledged for providing illustrations: Dr S. H. Lai (Fig. 13); Dr Gilbert Lau (Figs 14–16 and 28); Dr Chen Kugel (Fig. 63); Dr Matt Ryan (Fig. 70); Dr Rohan Ruwanpura (Figs 76–78); Queensland Health Scientific Services (Fig. 83); Dr Bob Hoskins, Government Medical Officer Services, Queensland (Fig. 86); Dr Donal Buchanan, Government Medical Officer Services, Queensland (Figs 84, 88, 90 and 92); the Victorian Institute of Forensic Medicine, Melbourne. Figure 150 was produced utilizing a computer program written by Dr Morris Odell.

The opinions and conclusions expressed by Dr Stephen Boos are those of the author and are not intended to represent the official position of the DoD, USAF, or any other governmental agency.

Contents

1   **Introduction to clinical forensic medicine** 1
    John A.M. Gall

2   **Crime scene and death** 3
    J. Jason Payne-James

3   **Post-mortem changes** 9
    J. Jason Payne-James

4   **External features** 21
    John A.M. Gall

5   **Injuries** 23
    John A.M. Gall

6   **Adult sexual assault** 61
    Elizabeth J. Culliford

7   **Child abuse** 69
    Stephen C. Boos

8   **Suicide** 99
    J. Jason Payne-James

9   **Motor vehicle accidents** 101
    John A.M. Gall

10 **Alcohol** 103
    John A.M. Gall

11 **Illicit drugs** 105
    Elizabeth J. Culliford

12 **Specimen collection** 119
    Elizabeth J. Culliford

13 **Blood stains** 125
    John A.M. Gall

14 **Photography** 127
    John A.M. Gall

Index 129

1 Introduction to clinical forensic medicine

Forensic medicine is a branch of medicine that interacts with the law, the judiciary and the police, where an extensive knowledge of medicine is essential to assist the legal process. The term is usually equated with forensic pathology and autopsies. In fact, forensic medicine covers the three areas of forensic pathology, forensic psychiatry and clinical forensic medicine.

Clinical forensic medicine is a relatively new term although the work it encompasses has been undertaken by doctors for centuries. Various terms have been used to describe practitioners of clinical forensic medicine including police surgeon, forensic medical officer, government medical officer and forensic medical examiner. More recently, and with the introduction of postgraduate training programmes in the discipline, the term *forensic physician* is used.

Unlike forensic pathologists, who generally deal only with the dead, forensic physicians have a broader role and also deal with the living. The actual role varies between jurisdictions but may include custodial (prison) medicine, traffic medicine (assessing suitability to drive), examination and interpretation of findings of adults and children alleging either physical or sexual assault or torture, assessment of alcohol and drug intoxication and withdrawal, assessment of mentally disturbed and intellectually impaired persons, assessment of fitness for detention in custody and interview by police, the collection of forensic samples, the conduct of intimate body searches, the investigation of deaths in custody, the examination of crime and death scenes (Figs 1 and 2), conduct autopsies, occupational health, and the provision of expert opinions in courts and tribunals.

Depending upon the specific tasks undertaken and the legal and forensic requirements of specific jurisdictions, the forensic physician requires appropriate equipment. Figure 3 shows an example of a forensic physician's 'doctor's' bag or forensic bag.

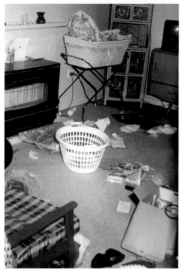

Fig. 1 Crime scene of alleged child abuse.

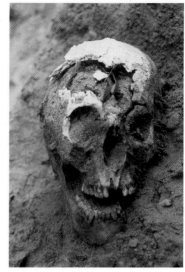

Fig. 2 Potential crime scene – unearthed skull.

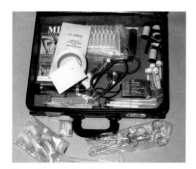

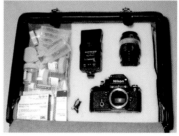

Fig. 3 Forensic kit with specimen collection material, medications and photographic equipment.

2 Crime scene and death

Crime scene

Edmund Locard introduced the theory of interchange in 1910, which stated that any contact between two objects will result in exchange of traces of material from one to another. It is this theory which lies behind much of today's investigative procedures for crime or suspected crime. The finding, recovery and scientific determination of traces of material provides the key links in the chain of evidence that may link a criminal to a specific crime. The investigation of crime is a complex and highly organized procedure that commences with the preservation of the scene of crime. Failure to follow strict protocols will allow the potential loss of evidence which may not be recoverable. In most jurisdictions a multidisciplinary support team will direct operations. This team may include uniformed police, detectives, crime scene examiners, forensic physicians (police surgeons), forensic scientists and forensic pathologists.

A scene of death is a clear example of a potential crime scene. Job titles and roles of the individuals involved will vary but the principles of investigation of a scene of death are the same as at any scene of crime. If a body is found, the first question to be answered is whether the death is suspicious or not. If it is at all suspicious (i.e. due to unnatural causes) the body should be examined by appropriately trained individuals such as forensic physicians and forensic pathologists. These doctors are able to assess the possible cause of death at a scene early on in an investigation, which may prevent unnecessary and expensive investigative work. However, in some cases the nature of the death will have to await an autopsy. An example of a suspicious death is the elderly woman found dead at home with bruising to her lower limbs (Fig. 4); these raised concerns for the non-medical investigators but were shown to be consistent with knocking into tables in the room (confirmed by her home help).

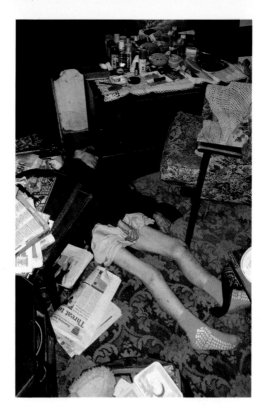

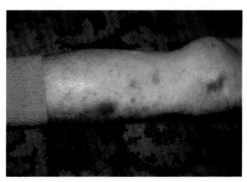

Fig. 4 Elderly woman, who had not been seen for 24 hours, with suspicious bruising to her lower limbs.

Categories of death

Deaths may be divided into five categories, some of which may be obvious at the initial assessment of the body.

Natural death

External factors are not usually involved and the death is due to a natural process or disease (e.g. myocardial infarction, cerebrovascular accident). Not all are immediately obvious (Fig. 5). This previously fit man was found dead in his workshop. Electrical tools were in place on the workbench, raising concerns of accidental electrocution. Autopsy revealed death to be due to a massive myocardial infarction.

Accidental death (sometimes known as misadventure)

A death is classed as accidental if it was unintentional but may have been caused by the deceased (e.g. autoerotic asphyxial death) or others (e.g. road traffic accidents). The case shown in Figure 6 is of a 60-year-old man found dead in the well of a block of flats. The photo was taken from a window that showed evidence of attempted entry (approx. 7 m from the ground). The man was a resident of the flats who, while drunk (blood alcohol 0.12%), had lost his keys, had tried to break into his flat, and fell. In the fall he sustained an occipital macerated laceration, a fracture and extradural haemorrhage.

Suicide

Suicide is death caused intentionally by the deceased through a deliberate act or acts intended to cause death (see also Chapters 5 and 8).

Homicide

Death due to someone else's specific actions. Death may have been the intended outcome or unintentional (where injury was the intent), in which case the term 'manslaughter' may be used in some jurisdictions. On a path near the body shown in Fig. 7 was a pile of clothes and literature suggesting suicide in a mentally disturbed person. However, investigation revealed that the man was the victim of abduction, torture and murder illustrating the need for caution in death assessment.

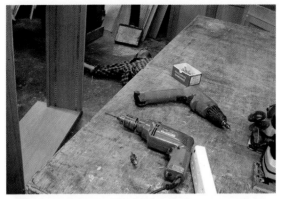

Fig. 5 Male found dead in his workshop with electrical tools on bench.

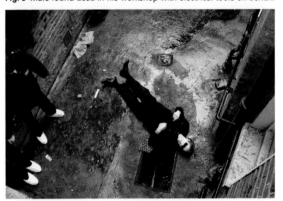

Fig. 6 Male found dead in well of a block of flats.

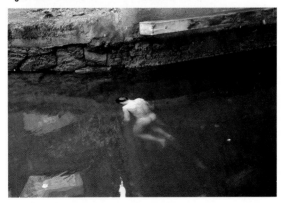

Fig. 7 Male found dead in a canal.

Undetermined

Classified as death where, despite full investigation (including the known events leading up to the death, and forensic and pathological examination), no clear cause of death can be identified.

Scene of death

If a scene of death is identified it is essential that as far as possible, within the constraints of safe working practices, the scene is preserved for preliminary examination. It is essential to secure a scene at the earliest opportunity; this is usually conducted by the police. An indoor scene is often more easy to secure than one outdoors, as there may be only one point of entry and the environment is generally constant. Outside (Fig. 8), weather changes, and the presence of water, animals and people may all affect the ability to secure the scene.

Crime scene examiners are trained to assess the scene and control movement (which must be documented in detail) in and out. Notes, sketches, photographic and video recordings enable a formal record of the scene to be made, which can be time and date coded. The environmental conditions (inside or outside) must be recorded (e.g. wind, temperature, rain, central heating, open fires, etc.). If the body is in water, the type of water, water temperature, tidal flows and presence of fish or other aquatic animals may be important. Evidence is recovered from the scene (e.g. fibres, glass, paint, soil, footprints, blood) which can be exhibited and analysed.

Additional specialist expertise may be brought to the scene (e.g. forensic physicians, forensic pathologists, forensic scientists). Each of these individuals must be directed through the scene by the crime scene examiner. Police firearms specialists were asked to attend the scene in Fig. 9 that was initially thought to be a suicide by gunshot to the head. The death turned out to be natural (a myocardial infarction), the gun was a non-working collector's item, and the apparent bleeding from the head was caused by putrefaction changes.

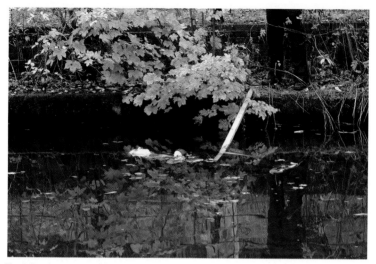

Fig. 8 Death scene requiring preservation of scene. The safety of investigators must be considered before recovery of the body.

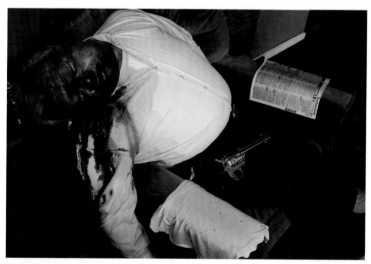

Fig. 9 Death scene with body displaying putrefactive changes.

3 Post-mortem changes

The external examination of the body at the scene (the 'locus') can reveal very important information with regard to time of death, manner of death, and site of death. In some circumstances, examination of the body at the scene is not practical. In these cases, as much information should be retrieved before removal to the mortuary. There are a number of specific changes that may occur in bodies after death as a result of decomposition, which may be unrelated to the manner of death, but may be influenced markedly by environmental factors. Some of the changes of decomposition may be present concurrently with others.

Hypostasis and livor mortis

Definition

Gravity accounts for one of the most important and significant post-mortem changes. Immediately after the cessation of blood circulation, blood will move into the capillaries and veins of dependent parts of the body. These capillaries and veins become relatively engorged and create a dark discoloration called lividity (livor mortis) or hypostasis (Figs 10–12). This appearance is evident in the surface tissues and all internal organs as early as 30 minutes after death and is maximal about 12 hours after death. Initially isolated patches develop, then become confluent. Skin colour is dependent on the ethnic origin of the individual and is generally of a purple–blue hue (Fig. 10), although reddish hues are not uncommon (Fig. 11). The presence of anaemia, or the loss of large amounts of blood in the immediate period before death, will result in a less marked colour change. A key feature of post-mortem hypostasis is that it is not present in those areas which were dependent, but pressed against a surface or an object after death – these areas are pale – due to 'post-mortem' sparing (Figs 10–12). The discoloration becomes fixed in the tissue after a few hours. Blanching of an area of hypostasis from thumb pressure indicates that fixing has not yet occurred (Fig. 12). ➡

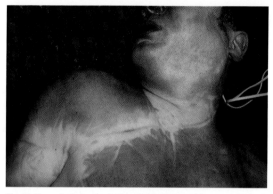

Fig. 10 Hypostasis in a male found dead jammed between his bed and the adjacent wall.

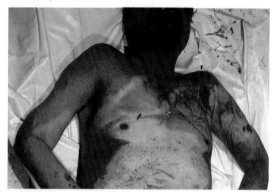

Fig. 11 Hypostasis with sparing in pressure areas.

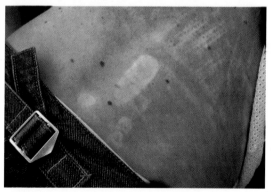

Fig. 12 Hypostasis with blanching discoloration from thumb pressure, showing that the hypostasis is not fixed.

Movement

The presence of an area of apparent hypostasis with a well delineated area of pale tissue is strongly suggestive that a body has been moved some time after the initial development of hypostasis, and may have substantial relevance in the investigation of a suspicious death. The presence of hypostatic changes on a non-dependent part should also raise the question of the body being moved. The colour change of simple post-mortem hypostasis must be distinguished from the pathognomonic colour change of acute carbon monoxide poisoning (cherry-red) (Fig. 13). Post-mortem hypostasis may be differentiated from bruising at autopsy, by confirming that the blood is retained within the vascular system rather than having extravasated into the adjacent tissues.

Adipocere

Definition

Adipocere formation (saponification) is a post-mortem change that takes place in the fatty tissue of the bodies. Adipocere is a greyish-white to brown, wax-like substance, which may become dry and brittle, composed of palmitic, oleic and stearic acids (Fig. 14). The odour is unpleasant and has variously been described as rancid, cheesy, earthy or ammonia-like. Adipocere develops as a result of hydrolysis of neutral fatty acids during putrefaction to form a mixture of the above-mentioned fatty acids and glycerol. These acids may be present in crystalline form. Adipocere appears to require moisture, either from the environment (extrinsic) or from the body itself (intrinsic). It is found in a wide variety of environmental conditions, including immersion in water and in damp graves. An acid pH environment is more likely to result in its formation. Adipocere can develop within a short period of several weeks or over months. Once developed, it is resistant to degradation and may be present for decades. It is this characteristic which allows identifiable facial features and recognizable wounds to be apparently retained (after saponification of fatty facial tissues) long after death. ➡

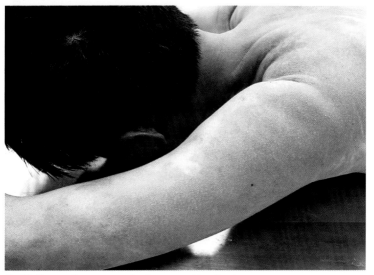

Fig. 13 Cherry-red appearance of carbon monoxide poisoning.

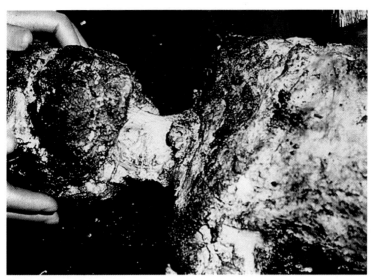

Fig. 14 Adipocere formation.

Rigor mortis

Definition

Rigor mortis describes the progressive stiffening of the muscles of the body. Immediately after death there is a period of flaccidity, followed by the development of rigor, which can commence within 30 minutes. This is followed by secondary muscular flaccidity after a period of time. Rigor develops as a result of a reduction in muscular ATP levels and the conversion of glycogen to lactic acid. Actin and myosin act together and solidify – creating the stiffness of rigor. It is sometimes (wrongly) used as an indicator of time of death. Rigor develops more rapidly when death has occurred after physical exertion, certain poisons, and electrocution. Care must be taken as rigor mortis may be confused with other post-mortem features that relate to special situations.

Cadaveric spasm

Cadaveric spasm (Fig. 15) is a condition in which the state of muscle contraction at the time of death is maintained into the post-mortem period, eventually ceasing as the changes of rigor mortis develop in other muscles. Anecdotally, cadaveric spasm appears to be most often present when death has been sudden, and particularly involves single groups of muscles (e.g. forearm and hand). Classic cases appear to occur when a drowning or falling person has attempted to pull themselves out of the water, or to arrest their fall by grasping at a plant on the bank or in the water or ground.

Heat rigor

Individuals who have died exposed to very high temperatures, causing muscle protein denaturation and coagulation, show heat rigor or heat stiffening (Fig. 16). Because of differing muscle bulks, the joints of upper and lower limbs stiffen in a position of flexion – which may give the characteristic 'pugilistic position' in death by fire.

Cold rigor

Extreme cold will cause cold stiffening – sometimes with the development of ice crystals. If the temperature is low enough at the time of death to allow freezing and cold stiffening or if cold rigor is present before true rigor mortis develops, then on thawing the body will develop rigor mortis in the same way as it would have done without freezing. ➡

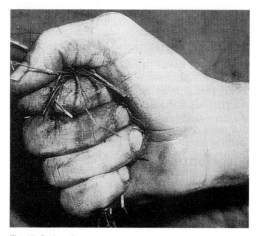

Fig. 15 Cadaveric spasm.

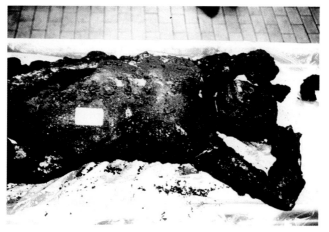

Fig. 16 'Pugilistic' appearance of a burnt body.

Putrefaction

Definition

In the absence of unusual or extreme environmental conditions or other external intervention, a body gradually undergoes a degenerative process caused by the presence of bacteria and endogenous enzymes. These cause an enzymatic breakdown of body tissues, which are manifest as a colour change, gas production and liquefaction within tissues (excluding bone) and hollow viscera. This process is known as putrefaction. Environmental and body conditions can either accelerate (hot climates, obesity, heavy clothing and sepsis) or slow down (cool climates) this process. Some environmental conditions delay or halt this breakdown process with resultant adipocere formation, or mummification. A range of organisms are present in life – with both respiratory and gastrointestinal systems being colonized – some pathogenic (perhaps associated with the cause of death), and some not.

Putrefactive changes

Decomposition may follow part or all of a sequence of events (the times of development depending upon the environment and body conditions). Initially, there may be a greenish discoloration of the lower abdomen and then the upper parts of the body (head, neck, shoulders). Swelling of the face (Fig. 17) occurs, followed by the development of 'marbling', generalized bloating and then skin slippage. The body at this point is usually a greenish-grey colour.

Colour

Skeletonization ensues over a variable period of time. The colour changes that occur are initially associated with haemolysis with local staining of tissues as a result of haemoglobin release. The colour changes can vary tremendously but are on a parallel with the variety of colour changes seen in bruise evolution (Fig. 18).

Gas formation

Gas formation may be manifest as bloating – most marked where the overlying skin is lax and unattached to underlying tissues (e.g. abdomen and scrotum). The presence of gas within the body cavities increases intracorporeal pressure, resulting in the outflow of bodily fluid and the products of putrefaction via orifices (especially the mouth and nose) (Figs 19 and 20).

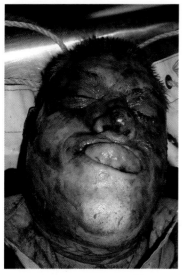

Fig. 17 Bloating and distension of facial features (note the tongue swelling and protrusion).

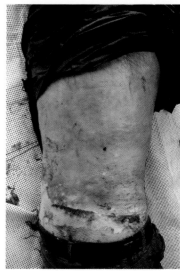

Fig. 18 Colour changes of putrefaction in a body that had been in the water for 1 week.

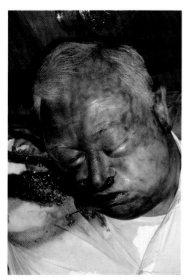

Fig. 19 Bloated head with putrefactive ooze from the mouth and nose.

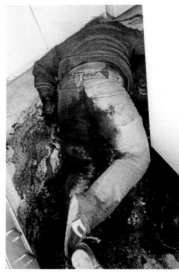

Fig. 20 Putrefactive ooze. The apparent blood is serosanguinous fluid.

Liquefaction	Tissue liquefaction occurs most rapidly in those organs with the least supporting connective tissue, but ultimately all soft tissues, skin, muscle, and internal organs will liquefy leaving the skeleton and dentition intact.
Marbling	Marbling (Fig. 21) describes one of the classic features of putrefaction, where bacteria colonize vascular channels and haemolyse blood. The classic branching pattern is initially a deepish red, outlining the superficial venous system. As putrefaction proceeds a greenish colour replaces this.
Skin slippage	Skin slippage is another stage of putrefaction, initially in the dependent areas of body where hypostasis is evident. The superficial layers of skin become elevated forming multiple, large, serous-filled bullae (Fig. 22). Whole segments of skin and hair-bearing skin may be mobile over the underlying tissues, and with gentle pressure may shear off in one piece (Fig. 23).
Maceration	Maceration is another form of putrefaction and is commonly used to describe the *in-utero* degeneration of an undelivered fetus. It should be noted, however, that this is not truly putrefaction as the process involved is one usually of septic autolysis. The sterile nature of the amniotic fluid results in elevation (as bullae) of superficial skin layers that detach (skin slippage) from underlying tissues. Maceration also describes the softening and apparent stretching of skin tissues, often seen in drowning, where there has been prolonged exposure to water. The pale, irregular appearance is caused by the detachment of upper skin layers from those that lie deeper and may be partial or complete, resulting in a 'degloved' appearance. At an early stage the term 'washerwoman's hands' may be used to describe the phenomenon (Fig. 24).

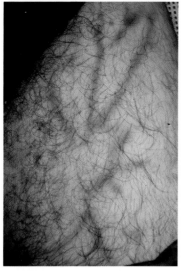

Fig. 21 Typical marbled appearance in the upper thigh of a drowned man.

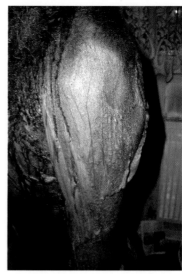

Fig. 22 Putrefactive changes of skin lift and fluid collection in large bullae on the shoulder.

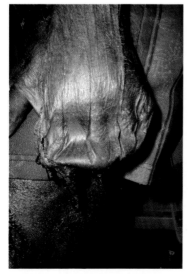

Fig. 23 Large fluid-filled bulla caused by slippage of the superficial layers of the skin.

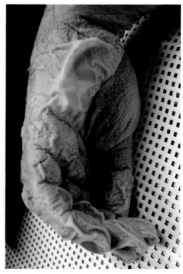

Fig. 24 Maceration of the hand of a drowning victim – 'washerwoman's hands'.

Animal and other predation

Animals (such as dogs, cats and rats), insects, crustaceans and fish may all create characteristic lesions after death (Fig. 25). Many of these may mimic wounds or specific injury types, the true origin of which may only be clarified at autopsy. For instance, water-borne insects (e.g. sea lice) in drowning victims can create lesions that mimic abrasions. Insects such as houseflies, blowflies and bluebottles may lay eggs on bodies. These hatch (the time being dependent on the species) and the larvae feed on the tissues locally (Fig. 26). The presence of flies, larvae and pupae (which should be collected and preserved, from both body and surroundings) may, with the expertise of a forensic entomologist assist in the determination of the time and the events surrounding death. Figure 27 shows the effects of animal predation: this man kept a cat, which was trapped with him in a room for 1 week after his death. Marks of the cat's dentition can be seen at the periphery.

Mummification

Mummification describes the process of decomposition that is accompanied by dehydration or dessication (Fig. 28). This results in dry, shrivelled, darkened tissues and organs that may be preserved for years – the best-known examples being those from Egyptian burial sites. Mummification is less common outside in temperate climates. Hair is retained and is often red in colour. Mummification may be seen in hidden infant deaths as there is only a small bacterial load, and so putrefactive changes may not develop rapidly. Mummification may take only a few weeks to develop, and may occur even more rapidly in deaths that have taken place inside, with dry central heating systems.

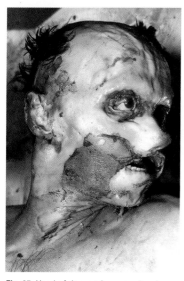

Fig. 25 Head of drowned person showing extensive damage caused by sea lice.

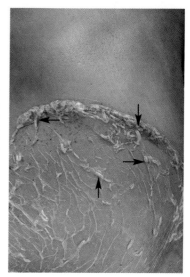

Fig. 26 Fly larvae (arrow) at the periphery of an area of skin lift.

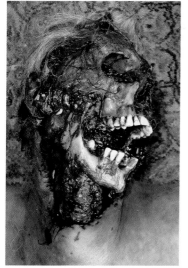

Fig. 27 Dramatic effects of animal predation.

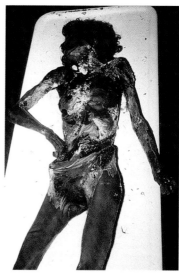

Fig. 28 Mummification.

4 External features

Clothing (see also Chapter 5) and ornaments worn and features identified on external examination of a person or body may provide important information regarding ethnic origin, past and present medical conditions and injuries, and give general impressions about the individual which all form part of the overall clinical picture. These features are also important to assist in the identification of an individual if necessary. When conducting a forensic examination, the documentation of these findings is essential and photography can be of considerable assistance. The clothing worn, its colour and the presence of any soiling or damage should be noted, as should the presence of any jewellery, body piercing and other ornamentation. In some cases, these items will be more extensively examined by forensic scientists in a laboratory setting. In addition, the person's ethnic origin (Fig. 29), height, weight, build, skin, eye and hair colour should be recorded. The presence of any visible medical condition (Fig. 30), recent and old scars, congenital abnormalities, striae and significant skin lesions, tattoos, and the presence or otherwise of circumcision should be noted. Also of importance is evidence of drug abuse (Fig. 31), the state of alertness of the individual and their personal hygiene.

Tattoos

Tattoos (Fig. 32) are important tools in the identification of a person or body due to their unique location and content. They remain visible in decomposing bodies and are thus of particular value. Tattoos may provide information about the person such as blood group, associations (individual and group) or interests. In some ethnic groups, tattoos are a prominent feature, although in Western countries, tattoos are becoming of less social significance.

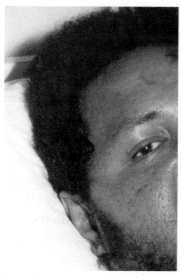

Fig. 29 External appearance of an individual provides information on ethnicity.

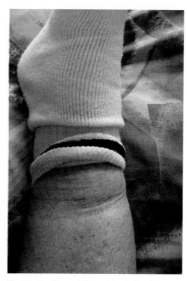

Fig. 30 Swelling of the ankles indicating an underlying medical condition.

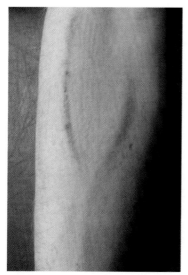

Fig. 31 Markings of intravenous drug use.

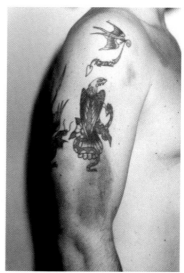

Fig. 32 Tattoos may be of great aid in identification.

Description and recording

Injuries are the 'bread and butter' of forensic medicine. Although the interpretation of these injuries may be best accomplished by forensic practitioners, their accurate description and documentation is the task of any competent doctor. Unfortunately, many doctors incorrectly describe, or fail to describe, injuries sustained by their patient. Within the medicolegal setting, this may lead to an injustice for the patient and a questioning of the doctor's competence. Injuries can be documented in narrative form but the most efficient and informative way is to use body charts (Fig. 33) or line drawings of a suitable size. Photography is a useful adjunct. The essential information to be recorded about any injury includes the nature of the wound, its location and appearance.

The nature of a wound provides information about the mechanism of injury. It is essential, therefore, that standard nomenclature be used. The principal injuries encountered include bruises, abrasions, lacerations, incisions, stab wounds, burns, fractures and penetrating injuries. More than one type of injury may co-exist.

The location of an injury is best described either on a body chart or in relation to fixed anatomical landmarks such as bony prominences or anatomical features (e.g. the eyes, mouth, nipples). All descriptions must relate to the standard anatomical position particularly when using terms such as lateral and medial.

When describing the appearance of an injury, the following, if relevant, should be documented: size (length, width and depth, preferably in millimetres); shape (regular, irregular, circular, ovoid, triangular, 'v' shaped); margins (regular, irregular, bruised, abraded); colour (and whether it is faint or dark); contents of the wound (e.g. foreign material or a scab); any evidence of healing. Ageing of injuries is notoriously inaccurate and should be approached cautiously.

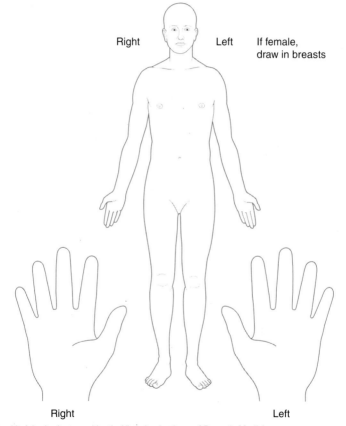

<table>
<tr><td colspan="2" align="center">Victorian Institute of Forensic Medicine</td></tr>
<tr><td>VIFM record number:
Date: Time:
Doctor's name:</td><td>Name: (or hospital label)</td></tr>
</table>

Right   Left   If female,
draw in breasts

Right   Left

Fig. 33 A body chart used by the Victorian Institute of Forensic Medicine.

Bruising

Definition

A bruise (contusion) is a focal area of discoloration due to the leakage of blood from ruptured veins and small vessels into the surrounding tissues and along anatomical planes.

Bruise appearance

The colour of a bruise varies but tends to be red, purple and grey and may change with time to include yellow, brown and green. There are a number of factors which may affect the appearance of a bruise:

Laxity of the tissue. In lax tissues (e.g. periocular tissues, scrotum) there is increased extravasation of blood and subsequent ease of bruising (Fig. 34) compared with areas of dense fibrous tissue (e.g. sole, palm).

Site of bruising. The vascular network varies from site to site, affecting the extent to which haemorrhage may occur. Tissue overlying bone tends to bruise more readily than more resilient areas such as the abdominal wall (Fig. 35).

Age. Children and elderly people bruise more easily than adults and increasing age is associated with delayed resolution.

Skin pigmentation. Bruises are more readily identified in non-pigmented or mildly pigmented skin.

Force of impact. The extent of haemorrhage will depend upon the force used, and the size and shape of the injuring object.

Diseases. Hypertension, scurvy, chronic alcoholism and coagulation disorders increase the extent of bruising.

Drugs. Drugs (e.g. steroids, anticoagulants) increase the extent of bruising.

Delayed presentation of bruises. Bruises may take a variable time (minutes to days) to appear.

Migration. Bruising may appear at a site remote from the point of injury (e.g. bruising may be seen in the periorbital region following injury to the forehead and/or scalp) (Fig. 36).

Other effects. Bruising can be affected by treatment and the nature of the injury sustained. ➡

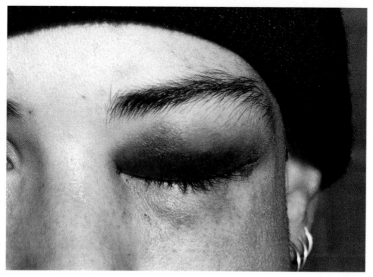

Fig. 34 Periorbital bruising.

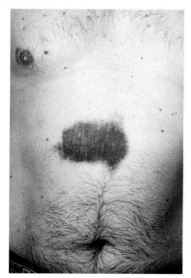

Fig. 35 Abdominal bruising.

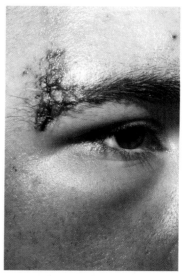

Fig. 36 Mild periorbital bruising following a laceration to the eyebrow.

Some bruises have features that are characteristic of their cause.

Petechial bruises. These are pinpoint areas of bruising (0.1–2 mm in diameter) resulting from venular rupture due to raised intravascular pressure. They are often seen on the conjunctiva, face and scalp after neck compression or following compression of the chest (e.g. crush injuries) (Fig. 37). They include 'love bites' and can be seen in a number of other non-forensic situations including prolonged cardiopulmonary resuscitation, bleeding diatheses and violent bouts of screaming, vomiting or coughing.

Imprint. Imprints are caused either directly by the implement used (Figs 38 and 100) or by an object placed between the skin and the blunt force (e.g. fabric; see Fig. 81, page 60).

Tramline. Following forceful contact with a linear object (e.g. a rod or a board) parallel linear bruises may appear separated by a central area of pallor (Fig. 39). This is referred to as a 'tramline' or 'railway line' pattern of bruising. Such bruising develops when a weapon strikes the skin, causing indentation of the tissue. There is tearing of the vessels at the edges of the indentation. At the centre, tissue compression occurs but the vessels tend to remain intact. On release of the pressure, blood flows back into the vessels and leakage occurs from the damaged vessels, forming the parallel bruises. However, such central sparing is not always present, particularly if there is underlying firm tissue such as bone.

Fingertip bruises. Firm finger grips on parts of the body may result in bruises that are round or oval. Characteristic locations include the neck in strangulation, medial aspect of the arms (Fig. 40), face or trunk of children (see Fig. 98, page 70), and medial thighs in sexual assault.

Bite marks. These are oval or curved bruises with central sparing, which may or may not be continuous (see page 38). ➡

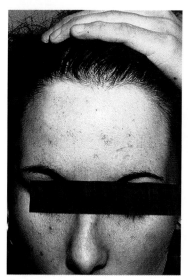

Fig. 37 Petechial haemorrhages on the forehead following neck compression.

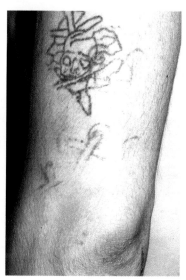

Fig. 38 Patterned bruise on the arm.

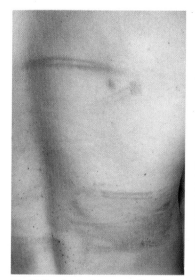

Fig. 39 Tramline bruising caused by a blow from a police baton.

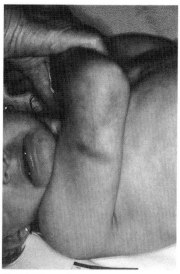

Fig. 40 Grip marks on the arm of a child.

The age of a bruise is frequently sought by investigators and the courts. Haemoglobin within the bruise breaks down to bilirubin and biliverdin and, logically, the colour of the bruise should change from red, violet or black to brown, green and yellow. This transition in colour is presented in older text books together with associated ages for the hues seen. However, recent research has shown that the age of a bruise cannot be determined accurately and that progressive colour change does not necessarily occur. This research has shown that:

- a bruise with a yellow border must be older than 18 hours (Fig. 41);
- red, blue and purple or black bruises may occur any time from 1 hour to resolution;
- a red appearance has no bearing on the age of a bruise; and
- bruises of identical age and cause on the same person may not appear as the same colour and may not change at the same rate.

In summary, the only reasonably certain aspect of the ageing of bruises is that a bruise with a yellow margin is 18–24 hours old or more.

Oedema, erythema and tenderness

Oedema (swelling) (Fig. 42), erythema (redness) and tenderness may be associated with trauma. There are, however, many other causes of these signs, unrelated to trauma. Although their presence is important and should be documented, they are not specific signs and their interpretation must be conducted with caution. Tenderness is particularly subjective in nature.

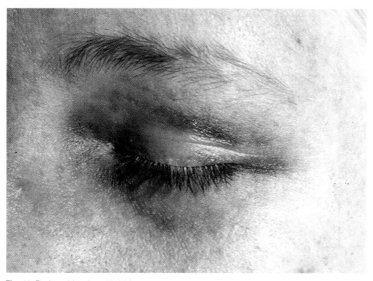

Fig. 41 Bruise older than 18–24 hours.

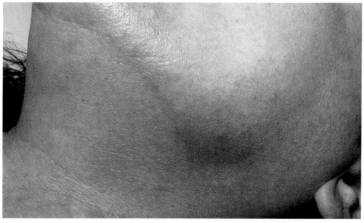

Fig. 42 Oedema of the angle of the jaw.

Abrasions

Definition

An abrasion (scratch, graze) is the result of blunt injury to the body causing disruption of the epidermis (outer layer of the skin).

Technically, an abrasion does not extend beyond the epidermis and does not bleed but, due to the convoluted nature of the papillary dermis and its vascular content, damage to the epidermis often does result in damage to the papillary dermis, with subsequent bleeding. The damage is caused by a combination of pressure and movement. It is an important injury in that it represents the site of contact with the implement or surface and may identify the direction of the force and the cause. Careful examination of the abrasion for skin tags (fragments of epidermis pulled towards the terminal end of the injury) may reveal the direction of the applied force (Fig. 43).

The many causes of abrasion include a blow or pressure from an object, bites, falls and being pulled along a surface (friction or carpet burns). Imprints may indicate the cause of the injury (radiator of a car, muzzle of a firearm). Of importance in sexual assaults and child abuse are fingernail abrasions and associated bruising. Fingernail abrasions may appear as straight or curved injuries. Where the tissue is grabbed and skin distortion occurs, these injuries may be inverted. Abrasions may occur on both the victim and assailant. In cases of strangulation, they may be present on the victim's neck due to attempts to release the assailant's hold (Fig. 44).

Ageing

Ascertainment of when an abrasion occurred is imprecise and will be modified by a number of factors including the extent of the injury, health of the individual, and the post-wound care. Early changes include the development of oedema and exudate on the surface. The margins become reddened within 12–18 hours (Fig. 45). Granulation tissue is evident at 24–72 hours and the tissue gradually heals.

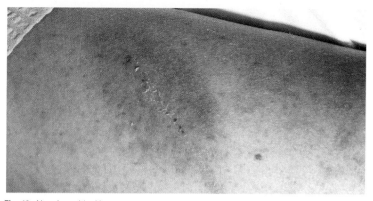

Fig. 43 Abrasion with skin tags.

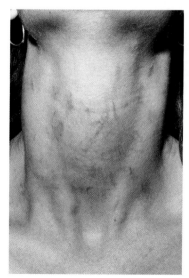

Fig. 44 Neck abraded by the victim's own fingernails.

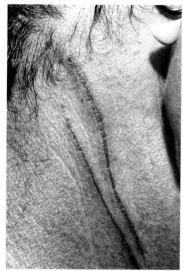

Fig. 45 Early healing abrasions.

Lacerations

Definition

A laceration is a tearing of tissue layers due to blunt trauma. A laceration of the skin is a tearing or splitting of the skin producing an injury which extends beyond the epidermis and into the underlying tissue layers.

Lacerations are distinct from incisions (Table 1) and the term should not be used to describe any 'cut' to the skin. There are a number of features, beyond the history of the injury, that will assist in distinguishing a laceration from an incision. Because of the nature of the crushing and tearing forces that have caused the laceration, its edges may be ragged, bruised, abraded, and inverted. An important feature of lacerations is the presence of bridging strands within the wound. These 'bridges' extend between the sides of the wound, particularly in the deeper aspects, and consist of fibrous strands, blood vessels and nerves. There is often profuse blood loss. Foreign material may be present within the wound.

Skin lacerations occur more readily on those parts of the body where there is an underlying firm base such as bone (Figs 46 and 47) but can occur in other locations (e.g. abdomen), depending upon the nature of the implement and force used. Lacerations may be caused by a variety of implements (e.g. bottles, bars) or as a result of part of the body coming in contact with a firm surface (e.g. falls, motor vehicle accidents). On occasions the cause of the laceration may be evident.

Ageing

A large number of factors (e.g. extent of injury, treatment and complications) will influence the rate of healing. All lacerations will heal and form a scar over a period of days to weeks. The absence of the features of healing will indicate a very recent laceration but once the healing process has begun, ageing becomes more imprecise.

Table 1 Features of lacerations and incisions

Feature	Lacerations	Incisions
Margins	• Ragged • Crushed • Abraded • Inverted • Bruised	• Regular • Not crushed • Usually not abraded • Everted • Usually not bruised
Foreign material	Yes	Not usually
Bridging strands	Yes	No

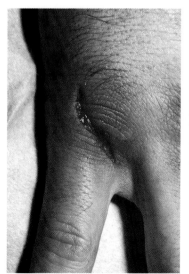

Fig. 46 Lacerated hand.

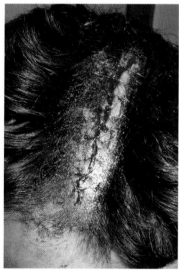

Fig. 47 Sutured laceration on the head caused by a baton strike.

Incised wounds

Definition

Incised wounds (slashes) are the result of sharp injury to the body resulting in regular, clean edges, the wound being longer than it is deep.

Incisions result from a tangential movement of the weapon (e.g. knife, razor, glass, scalpel) across the skin (Fig. 48). The wound may bleed profusely. Usually there is minimal damage to the surrounding tissues but this will depend upon any associated injuries. The margins tend neither to be bruised nor abraded. Deep structures may be involved and there may be foreign material in the wound, although this is less likely than in lacerations. There is a tendency for the wound to be deeper towards its origin and shallower towards its end but much depends upon the relative positions of victim and assailant, their respective movements at the time of injury and the anatomical location of the injury. With some incisions, abrasions may be present in continuity – due, for example, to the weapon tip being drawn across the skin after infliction of the 'cut'.

Incised wounds can be either accidental, the result of an assault or self-inflicted. In cases of assault, the incisions are often seen on the upper part of the body (especially the head and neck), on the ulnar aspect of the forearms and palmar surface of the hands and fingers. Incisions are often seen in cases of self-injury and tend to be located on the forearms and wrists. These incisions are often multiple and parallel and, in contrast with accidental and assault incisions, are frequently associated with tentative, superficial incisions and abrasions (Fig. 49).

Ageing

The clinical ageing of incisions is imprecise. Healing results in scab formation and erythema (12–24 hours) which intensifies with the formation of granulation tissue (24–72 hours).

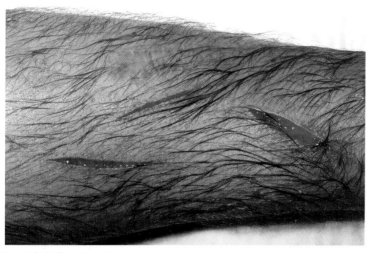

Fig. 48 Self-inflicted incised wounds on the forearm.

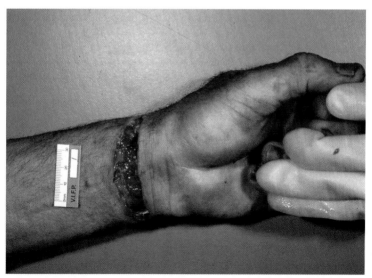

Fig. 49 Self-inflicted wrist incision with tentative markings and irregular depths.

Stab wounds

A stab wound is a penetrating injury, caused by a sharp or a blunt implement, where generally the depth of the wound is greater than its length.

Stab wounds are classified by some authors as a subclass of incised wounds. As the mechanism of injury is different from that of an incised wound and as non-sharp implements may be used to inflict these injuries, stab wounds are classified here as a separate wound type. Stab wounds may be accidental but are more often associated with assaults (Fig. 50), suicides (Fig. 51) and homicides. Suicidal stab wounds tend to be present over the anterior chest wall and abdomen and may be accompanied by tentative injuries such as superficial punctures. In cases of assault and homicide, defensive injuries may be present in addition to other injury types. Stab wounds can be caused by a large variety of weapons including knives, scissors, broken glass and screwdrivers.

The appearances of these injuries will vary according to the weapon used and any movement that may occur of the body or weapon while the weapon is being inserted or withdrawn. Appearance may provide information regarding the weapon type used. For instance, knives produce a wound that is usually slit-like or elliptical. If a knife with a single cutting blade and a thicker, blunt back is used, the angle made by the knife back may be split by contrast with the angle made by the cutting edge (Fig. 52). Once the weapon has been removed from the wound the length of the injury decreases and its width increases, due to the elasticity of the skin. Occasionally, where a knife has been driven in forcefully up to its hilt or handle, there may be bruising or abrasions of the skin. If blunt implements are used, there may be bruising at the margins and the skin may be split.

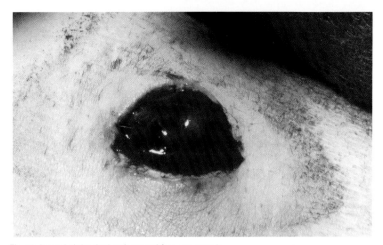

Fig. 50 Lateral abdominal stab wound from an assault.

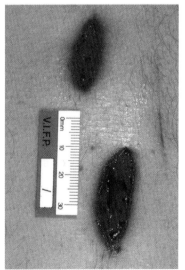

Fig. 51 Suicidal stab wounds to the abdomen.

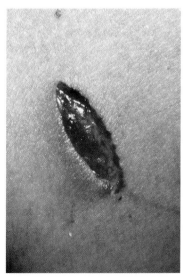

Fig. 52 Stab wound with split inferior corner.

Bites

Bites can be inflicted by humans (adult or child) or animals and the injuries caused may be one or more of bruising, abrasions, lacerations, punctures and amputations. Human teeth are arranged in a 'U' shape and the injury sustained from a human bite is usually distinctive, often appearing as oval or curved, opposing, U-shaped bruises with central sparing, which may or may not be continuous (Figs 53, 54 and 101).

   Although bites can occur at any site, the presence of these injuries on the neck and, more particularly, the breasts, buttocks and genitals, raises the possibility of sexual assault.

   'Love bites' (Fig. 55) are a special type of bite, in which the injury is due to suction on the skin, rather than actual biting, and causes the development of petechial bruising. These injuries can be seen in both consenting intercourse and sexual assault and tend to be located on the neck and breasts.

   Bite marks are forensically important and may provide identifying dental features of the offender, not unlike fingerprints. In forensic cases, these injuries should be examined by a forensic dentist. Where this is not possible, the injury must be carefully documented with measurements and, if possible, photographed. Recent bites should also be swabbed for DNA evidence.

Subconjunctival haemorrhage

The eye can receive a variety of injuries but the most common is a subconjunctival haemorrhage (Fig. 56). This is due to rupture of the small subconjunctival vessels and, in addition to direct blunt trauma, can occur from a bout of severe coughing or sneezing, screaming or neck compression.

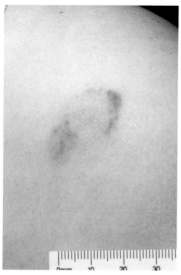

Fig. 53 Human bite mark.

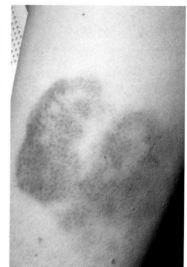

Fig. 54 Human bite mark.

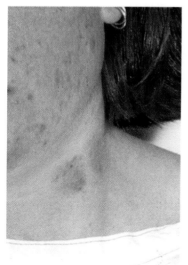

Fig. 55 'Love bite' on the neck.

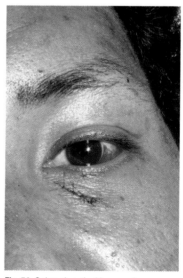

Fig. 56 Subconjunctival haemorrhage.

Fractures

In forensic medicine, fractures are generally encountered in cases of physical assault and are not uncommon in cases of suspected child abuse. In both adults and children, the extent of the physical force applied to normal bone will determine whether the fracture is complete or not. In children, greenstick (incomplete) fractures also occur.

Fractures in long bones may result from either direct or indirect force. Direct force results in a transverse or comminuted fracture at the point of impact with associated soft-tissue injury (Fig. 57). Indirect force results in a fracture at a point distant from the site of application of the force and soft-tissue damage at the point of fracture may not be evident (Fig. 58). The nature of the indirect force will modify the nature of the fracture. Twisting will cause a spiral fracture, bending a transverse fracture, and a combination of twisting, bending and compression will cause a short oblique fracture. Force applied to cancellous bone, including vertebrae and the skull, results in comminuted crush fractures. Avulsion fractures occur in circumstances where muscle action is resisted. In association with trauma to joints, a haemarthrosis may develop. When fractures are encountered, it is essential that associated soft-tissue injury is documented before any treatment.

Fractures may be detected clinically and confirmed radiologically. Not all fractures are evident initially but become apparent within 1–2 weeks. Isotopic bone scans may also be used to detect fractures but the presence of 'hot spots' must be cautiously interpreted as these merely represent sites of increased bone turnover (fractures, tumours, infections, physiological) and inflammation (arthritis, periostitis). 'Hot spots' must be correlated with plain films, computed tomography scans or magnetic resonance imaging. Fractures heal by callus formation.

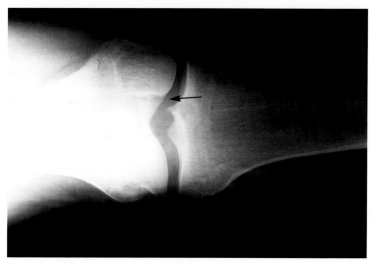

Fig. 57 Fracture (arrow) through the medial femoral condyle caused by a blow with a hockey stick to the bent knee.

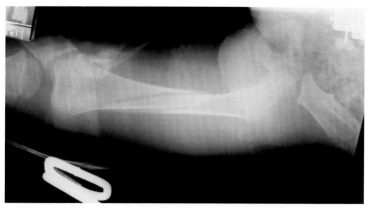

Fig. 58 Spiral fracture of the femur, allegedly following a fall from a bicycle.

Burns

Burns can occur accidentally or intentionally. They result in tissue damage which varies depending upon the mechanism and extent of injury. Mechanisms for thermal injury include the following:

- *Scalds* caused by hot fluids, which result in areas of erythema and blistering (Fig. 59).
- *Contact burns* due to direct contact of the hot implement with the skin (e.g. cigarette burns, branding) (Figs 60, 111 and 112). The burns often have features shaped like the implement with well-defined edges and a uniform depth of injury. Cigarette burns may have a crater-like appearance.
- *Fire* results in a variety of injuries including singed hair, areas of erythema, blistering, skin loss and charring. Incineration can occur; this may generate artefacts that mimic injury including splits in the skin, amputations and haematomas.
- *Electrical burns* result in injuries with minimal or no erythema to extensive and severe burns (Fig. 61). In cases of electrocution, electrical entry points may be identified; these often consist of one or more intact or collapsed (raised rim with a central pit) blisters or keratin nodules (brown–yellow fused keratin surrounded by pale skin).
- *Radiation burns* from periods of exposure result in areas of erythema and blistering.
- *Chemical burns* caused by solid or liquid chemicals may result in areas of erythema and blistering.
- *Friction burns* are due to the skin being dragged across a surface (e.g. carpet burns) (Fig. 62) or a surface rubbed across the skin. This may result in areas of abrasion, which tends to be more marked over bony prominences.

Clothing worn by an individual will modify the extent of burns, as will any treatment received.

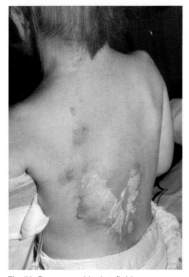
Fig. 59 Burn caused by hot fluid.

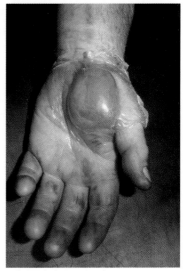
Fig. 60 Contact burn from hydronic heating.

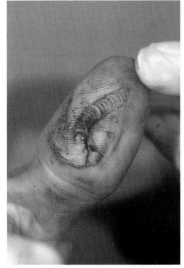
Fig. 61 Electrical burn from a hair dryer.

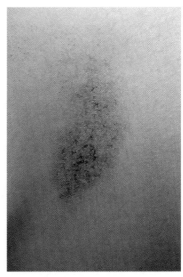
Fig. 62 Carpet friction burn.

Projectile injuries

Injuries from projectiles (e.g. crossbows, captive-bolt guns, air weapons, home-made weapons, missile fragments from explosions) will depend upon the type of missile and its associated force. For low-velocity projectiles (up to 340 m s^{-2} or 1100 ft s^{-2}) the tissues may be directly lacerated or crushed with secondary damage to adjacent structures. Tertiary damage may result from firm tissue fragments (e.g. bone and cartilage) that are displaced and produce subsequent damage within the body. High-speed projectiles (exceeding the speed of sound) cause injuries due to compression and cavitation.

Rifled weapons

Projectiles from these weapons may cause both entry and exit wounds. Small-calibre bullets (0.22) often do not exit from the body.

Entry wounds

Contact. Circular wound. There may be a muzzle mark, bruising and burning of skin and hair (Fig. 63).

Close range (up to about 20 cm). Circular wound with some smoke soiling, powder burns and skin and hair burning. The edges of the wound are inverted and there is an abrasion collar (Fig. 64).

Longer ranges. Up to 1 m, smoke soiling, burning and powder tattooing may be present. Beyond 1 m the entry will have only an abrasion collar. Bullets hitting tangentially will cause an eccentric abrasion collar.

Exit wounds

These tend to be larger than entrance wounds and usually consist of irregular lacerations and holes with everted, unabraded and non-bruised margins. Additional exit wounds may be due to the exit of fragmented bone and cartilage from the body. ➡

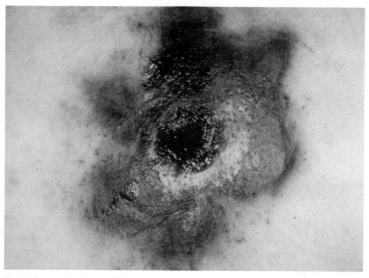

Fig. 63 Contact discharge of M16 with burns, soot from fire suppressor and entry hole.

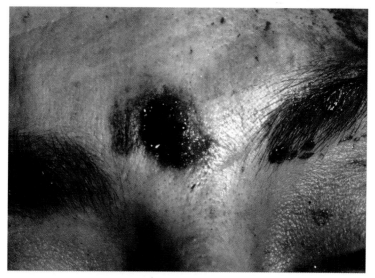

Fig. 64 Tangential near contact wound from a .22 rifle.

Smooth-bore weapons (shotguns)

The shotgun is the most common smooth-bore weapon and is generally either a 12-gauge with a diameter of about 19 mm or a 410 with a diameter of about 11 mm. The appearance of the wound will depend upon the discharge distance.

Entry wounds

Contact.   The wound is a neat, circular, abraded hole, with a diameter equivalent to approximately the size of the muzzle (Figs 65 and 66). There is usually some smoke soiling. The tissues within the wound may be pink due to the presence of carbon monoxide in the discharged gases. If the weapon is discharged over underlying bone, there may be splitting of the skin. With a double-barrelled shotgun, a muzzle imprint of the second barrel may be evident.

Near (up to 15–20 cm).   Wounds are similar to contact wounds but without evidence of a muzzle mark. Burning of the skin and singeing of hairs may be seen. Burning flakes of propellant may also be present causing burning to the surrounding skin.

Short range (20 cm–2 m).   Smoke soiling may still be present and powder tattooing will continue in decreasing amounts up to about 1 m. Wads may be seen either in or near the wound but these rarely travel more than 2 m. The entry hole will change with increasing distance, becoming scalloped or rat-hole-like at about 1 m.

Longer range.   The shot spreads progressively with the formation, at distances of 2–3 m, of satellite pellet holes around a central wound. At longer ranges (20–30 m) there is uniform peppering of the shot.

Exit wounds

Unusual but this will depend upon the nature of the shot and site of the body hit (Fig. 67).

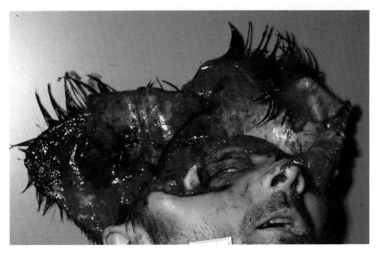

Fig. 65 Contact wound to head caused by 12G shotgun.

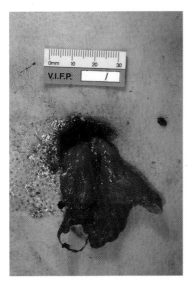

Fig. 66 Near contact shotgun injury to chest.

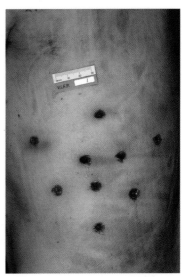

Fig. 67 Exit wounds of shotgun pellets.

Self-inflicted injuries

Self-inflicted injuries are regularly seen in forensic medicine and are not uncommon in other areas of medicine, particularly in emergency and psychiatric departments. The young female presenting with either multiple incised injuries to her wrists or a deliberate drug overdose resulting from an emotional upset or depression is not uncommon. In general, there are five types of self-inflicted injuries:

- those intended to result in death (Fig. 68);
- those where the individual is making a 'cry for help';
- self-inflicted wounds, where the injury is the goal (e.g. cultural practices, body piercing and ritualistic mutilation) (Fig. 69);
- injuries caused by people with psychiatric disorders (Fig. 70) including Munchausen's syndrome;
- injuries that are designed for a secondary gain.

In forensic medicine, all groups of self-inflicted injury are encountered. Those inflicted for secondary gain, however, regularly present within the forensic setting and it is this group that is discussed further here. The types of gain for this group vary considerably but include claims for compensation, revenge, to escape prosecution, to gain some form of advantage in adverse situations such as in the custodial system, and to divert attention. This group fit within the definition of malingering in DSM-IV as 'the intentional production of false or grossly exaggerated physical or psychological symptoms, motivated by external incentive such as avoiding military duty, avoiding work, obtaining financial compensation, evading criminal prosecution, or obtaining drugs'. ➡

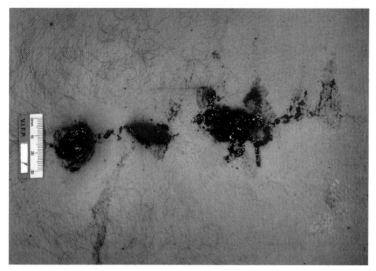

Fig. 68 Suicidal stab wounds to abdomen.

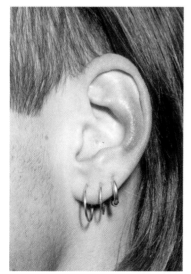

Fig. 69 Ear piercing.

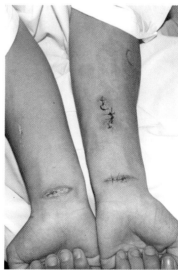

Fig. 70 Self-inflicted incisions in a psychiatric patient.

Self-inflicted injuries (excluding those where severe mutilation is intended such as with some psychotic patients and where death is the intended outcome) include the following features (Figs 71–73):

- usually not fatal;
- tend to be superficial;
- often multiple and parallel;
- tend to be of a single injury type;
- generally consist of abrasions or incisions rather than bruises or lacerations;
- often all injuries are of similar severity;
- usually involve non-vital structures such as the cheeks, forehead, chest, abdomen, and upper and lower limbs but tend not to involve the eyes;
- present on accessible sites (i.e. a right-handed individual will preferentially injure the left side of the body);
- overlying clothing is often spared; and
- an absence of defensive injuries.

An incorrect diagnosis in these cases may have significant consequences in the justice system, particularly for the accused. Thus, a thorough history (which may raise suspicions as the injuries are incongruous with the allegations) and physical examination are essential, together with the complete documentation of the findings and, if possible, photography of the injuries. Depending upon the case history, the clothing worn at the time of the alleged occurrence of the injuries should be examined, if possible with the subject wearing them. Sometimes it is important for the subject to demonstrate the position they and their alleged assailant were in when the injuries were sustained. In addition, an inspection of the crime scene may be helpful to the interpretation of the injuries. In many circumstances, it can be very difficult on medical grounds alone to determine whether the injuries are incontrovertibly the result of self-infliction.

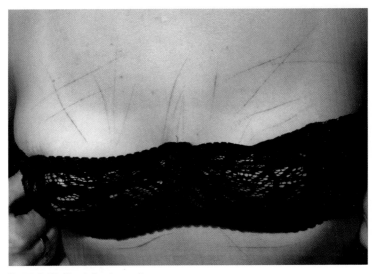

Fig. 71 Self-inflicted abrasions to breast.

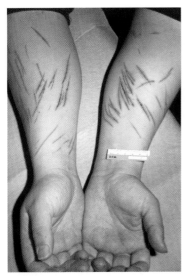

Fig. 72 Self-inflicted abrasions and incisions to forearms.

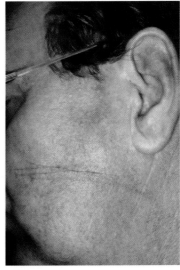

Fig. 73 Self-inflicted abrasions to the cheek.

Defensive injuries

Defensive injuries occur in an attempt at self-protection from implements used during an assault.

The presence or absence of defensive injuries may assist in determining the legitimacy of an allegation of assault: their absence does not, however, disprove such an allegation. Defensive injuries generally consist of one or more of bruises, abrasions, lacerations and incisions. Other types of injuries (e.g. burns, bites, fractures) may occur but are less common. There are three general locations where defensive injuries are found:

Upper limbs. It is a natural response to use the upper limbs to protect the upper part of the body from blows with an implement, particularly when upright but also when on the ground and in the fetal position. In doing so, the extensor and ulnar aspects of the forearms and hands in particular become exposed to injury (Fig. 74). Similarly, attempts are sometimes made to grab the offending weapon. If the weapon has an edge, such as a knife, injuries may be present on the palmar aspects of the hand and fingers (Fig. 75). These injuries should be examined to ascertain the nature of the injury, whether the wounds on the fingers are continuous or the result of more than one injury.

Thighs. When the victim is standing and a blow is being directed to the lower part of the body, it is natural to turn the thigh towards the blow. This may result in injuries (usually bruises) on the lateral aspects of the thighs.

Neck. During some attacks, the victim may be grasped around the neck. In an attempt to release the grip, the victim may sustain bruising and abrasions as a result of their own fingernails being forced between the compressing object and the skin of their neck (see Fig. 44 p. 32).

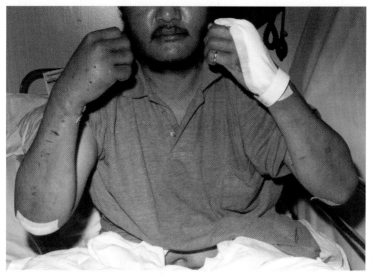

Fig. 74 Defensive injuries on forearms and hands.

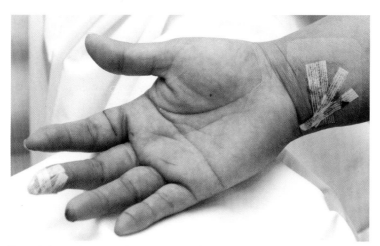

Fig. 75 Defensive incised injuries caused by a knife.

Torture

Torture is not uncommon and its infliction may result in both physical (internal and external) and psychological injuries. The means used for torture are many and varied with some characteristic of particular countries or cultures. As with all injuries and ailments, those due to non-torture need to be distinguished from those resulting from torture. In many cases, this is assisted by a detailed history, which may provide information as to the extent and cause of the initial injury, treatment and the healing process.

Injuries may only present for medical examination during or after healing and must be carefully documented. Internal injuries may not be evident without laboratory or imaging investigation. Damaged joints and muscle groups and fractures may present with one or more of pain, restricted mobility, loss of strength and loss of bulk. Externally, the principal findings may be of healing injuries or scars. These injuries result from varied causes.

- Ligatures around the wrists and ankles (Fig. 76).
- Beating or whipping tend to involve the back and buttocks. The scars formed will depend upon the weapon used which may include, whips, sticks, hoses, truncheons and belts (Figs 77 and 78). The injuries may be linear or criss-cross. Buckles may leave a patterned scar.
- Burning or branding with an object may leave a patterned scar. Burns with cigarettes may leave a circular scar and, in more severe burns, an indented scar.
- Electrical burns rarely leave scars but sometimes leave white circular scars or groups of red, punctate marks. The preferred sites for these injuries include the nipples, scrotum and penis.
- Stab wounds and incisions.
- Damage to or removal of fingernails and toenails.
- Amputations – particularly of the ears, digits and genitalia.

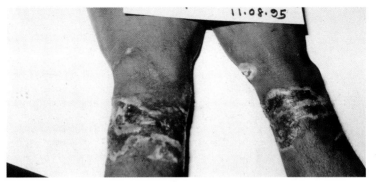

Fig. 76 Healing wrist injuries following binding and suspension from a beam.

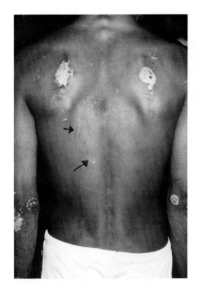

Fig. 77 Healing injuries to back and elbows, including tramline bruising (arrows), following an assault.

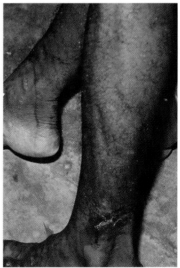

Fig. 78 Healing lacerations to ankles following an assault with clubs and a rubber hose.

Weapons

The weapon allegedly used in an assault may be available for comparison with the injury sustained (Figs 79 and 80). This is particularly useful with patterned injuries. The medical examiner in some cases may be able to assist in advising whether the weapon was a likely cause of the injury or injuries sustained by the victim.

Care must be taken when handling the alleged weapon, particularly if seen before examination by the forensic scientists. It should be examined separately from the victim and contamination must be avoided. Some weapons are potentially infective.

When examining the weapon, the features that would match with the injuries should be documented including the following, as appropriate:

- dimensions of the weapon;
- composition of the weapon (e.g. metal, wooden)
- description and measurements of the patterns (photographs of the weapon and patterns are ideal but must include a scale);
- number and nature of cutting or other edges;
- sharpness of tips and edges;
- any unusual features;
- the presence and shape of the guard or hilt;
- whether intact or broken or bent;
- the presence of blood-like stains or other material.

Handcuffs

Handcuffs, although not necessarily a weapon, may leave non-continuous red marks about the wrists. Abrasions, joint and nerve injuries may also occur if handcuffs are used inappropriately or the detainee tries to free himself.

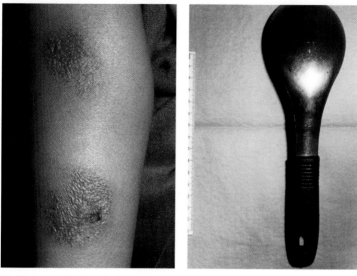

Fig. 79 Burns to leg from the heated spoon shown.

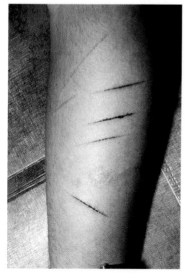
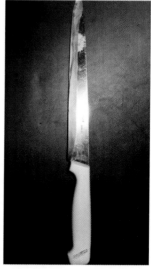

Fig. 80 Self-inflicted abrasions and incisions from the knife shown.

Clothing

Not all allegations of an assault are legitimate and the clothing worn at the time of the alleged crime may assist with the medical interpretation of the injuries sustained. On such occasions, the subject should be examined as soon after the alleged incident as possible and wearing the clothes worn during the incident. If this is possible the clothing can be examined separately. Formal assessment of any clothing is the preserve of the forensic scientist.

There are several occasions with regards to the documentation and interpretation of injuries where an examination of the clothing (victim's and/or offender's) may be beneficial.

- Where the history of the alleged assault does not match with the appearance of the individual (e.g. assaults occurring in a dirty or muddy environment but there is no evidence of the environmental material on the clothes worn at the time).
- Where there are patterned injuries. The patterns may originate not from a weapon but from the clothing interposed between the source of force and the skin (Fig. 81).
- Where expected injuries are either absent or not as extensive as expected. Some clothing may be protective and modify the appearance of the resultant injury (e.g. woollen clothing protecting from hot-water burns).
- Where wounds may have been self-inflicted. A feature of self-infliction may be the preservation of the clothing worn at the time of infliction – the site of injury is exposed and then covered with the clothing again after the injury has been inflicted. Alternatively, either the location of the injury on the body does not coincide with the anatomical site of the injury or the damage to the clothing is inconsistent with the mechanism of injury (Fig. 82).

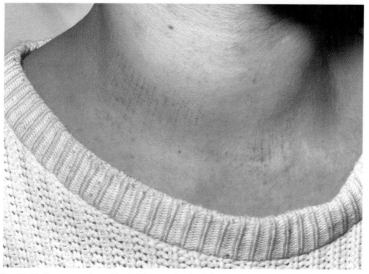

Fig. 81 Neck compression with clothing causing bruising.

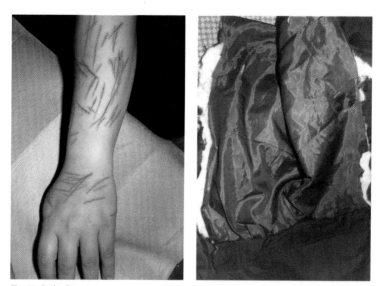

Fig. 82 Self-inflicted abrasions and incisions on forearms, but the opened sleeve (right) worn at the time of injury is not apparently damaged.

The optimal response to an individual who has been sexually assaulted requires the cooperation and coordination of a number of agencies and individuals including police, medical, counselling and legal personnel. The service provided should focus on the individual's needs ensuring safety, privacy and confidentiality. The response should be timely and non-judgemental, sensitive to the individual in terms of language, culture, age, disability, gender, sexuality and location. The care provided should encourage the individual's sense of personal control and respect and support their informed decision at every stage of the process.

Medical response

The medical response should be provided by healthcare professionals who have appropriate training, expertise and support. The main aspects of this response are safety of the individual, choice, information and consent, and medical, psychosocial and forensic issues.

The expected acute response of the doctor should include:

- documentation, treatment and interpretation of injuries;
- provision of post-exposure prophylaxis for sexually transmitted infections;
- provision of post-coital contraception;
- completion of the forensic examination with the taking of medical evidence samples using appropriate materials/kits for the jurisdiction (Figs 83 and 84); and
- provision of follow-up care or referral to other health services for follow-up care.

Consent

Informed consent for the forensic examination and disclosure of any information to the police and courts is necessary. A chaperone should be present at the examination. ➡

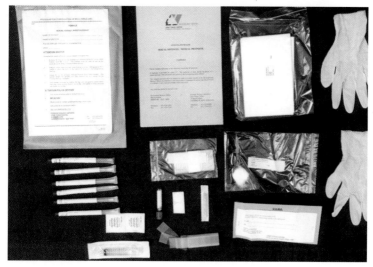

Fig. 83 Sexual assault investigation kit.

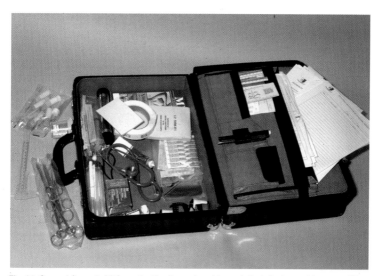

Fig. 84 General forensic kit for collecting forensic evidence in jurisdictions without specific kits.

History	When performing the forensic examination, a full history should be taken from the victim including details of current and past medical, surgical and psychiatric conditions, current medications (including contraception), and a brief history of the alleged assault. Of note regarding the assault is any orogenital contact, ejaculation and where the semen landed, positions used and any force or threat of force used. It is important to note any use of drugs, any defence used (such as biting or scratching), any injuries sustained, however minor, and how they were sustained. Other information sought should include previous intercourse within seven days, whether a condom was used during the assault and whether the victim has bathed or showered and changed clothing since the assault.
Examination	A full clinical examination is then performed after the victim has undressed on a clean drop-sheet (paper sheet) and has put on a clean hospital gown. Any items of clothing worn at the time of the assault should be placed individually in clean paper bags, labelled and sealed. The police may take some or all of this clothing as evidence. A complete external examination of the victim is conducted, preferably with the examining doctor wearing latex gloves. All injuries should be fully documented. Careful examination of the mouth may reveal abrasions or lacerations on the gingival or buccal mucosa (Fig. 85). Blunt force injuries to the face may result in a periorbital haematoma (Fig. 86) or tender lumps on the scalp. Bruising and abrasions to the neck (caused either by the assailant or by the victim trying to release the assailant's grip) (Figs 44 and 87) associated with sub-conjunctival (Fig. 88) and facial petechial haemorrhages (Fig. 37) may follow attempted strangulation. There may be bruising behind the ears or lacerations to the ear lobes if earrings have been forcibly removed. Blows to the ear may rupture the tympanic membrane. ►

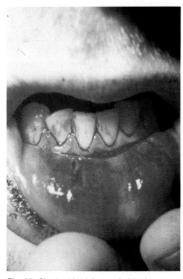

Fig. 85 Gingival bruising and abrasion.

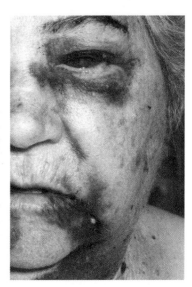

Fig. 86 Facial injuries in an elderly patient due to assault.

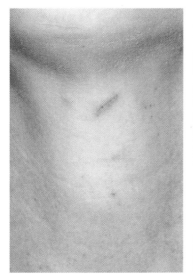

Fig. 87 Abrasions to neck following attempted strangulation.

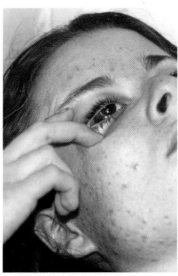

Fig. 88 Subconjunctival haemorrhage following attempted strangulation.

Bite marks may be found anywhere but are more commonly found on the neck and breasts. These may be bites caused by teeth (Figs 53, 54 and 89) or suction bruises ('love bites'; Fig. 55). Bruises from blunt trauma can be found anywhere on the body and may be due to the assailant hitting the victim or the victim falling against a hard object such as furniture or part of a car. There may be fingertip bruising on the upper arms or shoulders (Fig. 90) or abrasions or bruises to the wrists if the victim has been held forcibly.

Abrasions may be caused by the assailant (such as scratches with nails or from the tip of a knife) or the environment. The back, buttocks, elbows and knees are areas that may show minor injuries such as irregular abrasions sustained from the ground/floor (Figs 91 and 92) or other firm objects where the assault occurred.

Genital examination

The genital area should be examined after changing gloves. The inner upper thighs may show oval or round fingertip bruises similar to those often found on the upper arms or wrists. In female victims, the genital examination should include the mons pubis, labia majora, labia minora, vaginal introitus, posterior fourchette, hymen, urethra, clitoris, perineum, perianal skin and anus. The examination is performed with the patient in the supine position then in the left lateral position. Abrasions, bruising, lacerations, bites, redness, tenderness and swelling should all be noted.

Speculum examination

A speculum examination is usually performed to exclude vaginal or cervical injuries and the presence of foreign bodies. It also allows the collection of an uncontaminated cervical os and/or a high vaginal swab to be taken for semen detection.

Male victims

In male victims, the genital examination includes penis, foreskin (if uncircumcised), scrotum, testes, perianal skin and anus. Proctoscope examination is usually performed if anal intercourse is suspected, to exclude rectal injuries, foreign bodies and to allow an uncontaminated rectal swab to be taken for semen (both males and females). ➡

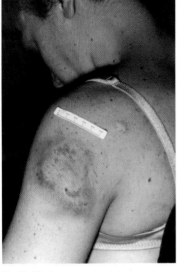

Fig. 89 Bite to arm.

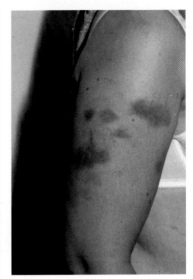

Fig. 90 Fingertip bruising to arm.

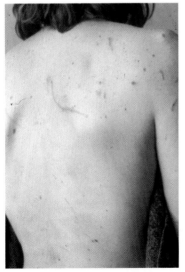

Fig. 91 Abrasions from vegetation.

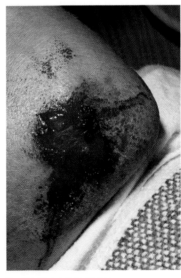

Fig. 92 Abrasion to elbow.

The forensic specimens collected will depend on the history given by the victim (see Chapter 12). The offender's spermatozoa may be isolated from the victim's cervical os, vaginal, vulval, oral, anal/rectal and skin swabs; the offender's buccal cells may be isolated from a bite or an area licked; fingernail scrapings may contain the offender's blood or epithelial cells; there may be stray hairs from the offender on the victim.

Bites may also be matched to an offender. Blood and urine taken from the victim may reveal drugs or alcohol, perhaps administered to facilitate the assault. The victim's vaginal or rectal cells may be isolated from swabs taken from the suspect's penis.

The issue of consent given by a victim for intercourse remains the most difficult to prove or disprove in court. Interpretation of the presence of injuries must be cautiously approached. The presence of injuries, including genital injuries, may suggest that the act was non-consensual. However, it needs to be remembered that injuries may occur in consensual intercourse – it depends upon how intercourse, and the sexual act in general, was conducted. Only 30% of victims of a sexual assault have physical or genital injuries, with abrasions, bruises and lacerations being the most common. Serious and potentially life-threatening injuries occur in 2–5% of victims and injuries causing death in about 1%. Injuries from forcible restraint (e.g. rope burns) and evidence of torture (e.g. cigarette burns) (Fig. 93) may be evident but can be either consensual or non-consensual. Self-inflicted injuries (Fig. 71) may cause some confusion: they may be easy to diagnose by their nature and position (Figs 94 and 95) or the history does not correspond with the findings. Overall, in about 50–60% of victims the physical examination may be normal. However, the absence of injuries, especially genital injuries, does not exclude non-consensual intercourse having taken place.

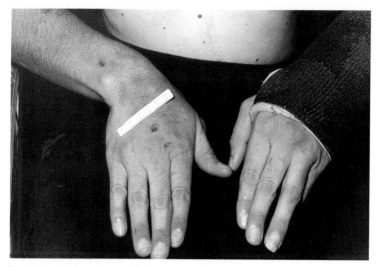

Fig. 93 Cigarette burns to upper limb.

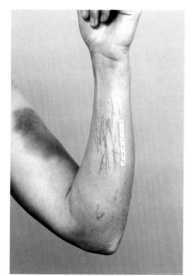

Fig. 94 Self-inflicted injuries to forearm.

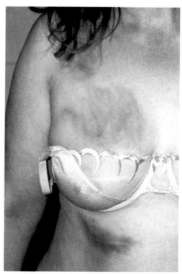

Fig. 95 Self-inflicted bruising to breast and ribs.

Physical abuse

The initial phase in evaluating child physical abuse is recognizing the possibility that a child's injuries may be inflicted. Patterns in the visible injuries, findings strongly associated with abuse, and inconsistencies between the given history and the actual injuries will alert the examiner to the possibility of abuse.

Cutaneous trauma

Marks on the skin may present a picture of what caused them. In the case of bruises, a positive or negative image of the impacting object may appear, as blood vessels are crushed under the area of contact, or stretched and torn at the margins of impact. A bruise becomes apparent when blood released from the injured vessels rises into the visible layers of the skin. Because migration of blood is necessary for deeper injuries to become visible, bruises may be delayed in presentation, or only visible if the injured part is incised at autopsy.

Patterned injuries

The hand is the most readily available weapon for injuring a child, and hand marks are commonly seen abusive injuries. Open-handed slap marks present with confluent lines of petechiae outlining the fingers of the hand. With time the individual petechiae blur and blend together. This may appear as parallel or diverging rays, loops or ladders (Figs 96 and 97). Forceful grabbing of a child may cause bruising when the fingertips are driven into the soft tissues. The oval bruises that result are non-specific, but the arrangement of three or four such bruises in an arc of appropriate size may be recognized as a grip mark (Fig. 98). ➡

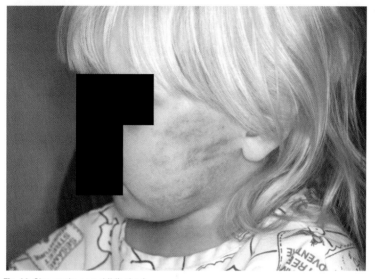

Fig. 96 Slap marks on a child's cheek.

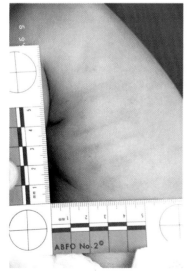

Fig. 97 Older slap mark on a child's thigh.

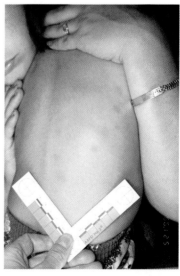

Fig. 98 Grip marks on a child's back.

Other common household objects are frequently used to strike children. Switching or caning with a lightweight stick, and whipping with a belt or loop of electrical cord (Fig. 99), are widely used methods of punishment. Other household objects may be impulsively grabbed, and used to strike a child (Fig. 100).

Lightweight objects with proportionately high surface area dissipate their energy superficially. Under such circumstances the dermal capillary bed is compressed under the object, and stretched along its margins. The stretched capillaries may break, creating confluent petechiae outlining the object. These injuries are visible immediately, or within a few hours of infliction. With time the individual petechiae become indistinct, and merge into the larger pattern of the bruise. In darkly pigmented individuals, these marks are frequently preserved beyond the duration of bruising as hyperpigmented marks. The same weapons may cut or tear the skin. A raised scar or smooth hypopigmented skin may then remain within the outlines of the object.

Impacts with more concentrated force will make more penetrating contact, crushing vessels in deeper tissues. Such damage is not immediately visible. Released blood will diffuse through the tissues, and may become visible at the skin's surface hours to days after injury. This same process of diffusion may result in indistinct bruise shape and margins, and displacement of the bruise from the original site of injury. The appearance of a 'black eye' a day after a child strikes his or her forehead is a classic example of this last phenomenon.

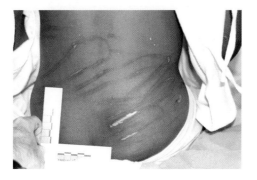

Fig. 99 Loop of cord marks on a child's back.

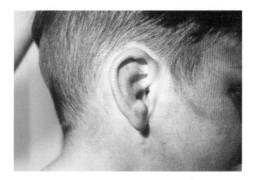

Fig. 100 (a) Imprint of a shoe on a child's face, ear and head.

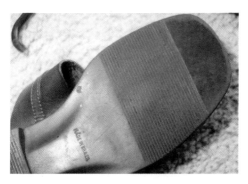

Fig. 100 (b) Ridged sole of the shoe used to strike the child.

Not all bruises arise from a blow. Crushing, stretching and chafing of the skin may also cause blood vessel rupture, and thus bruising.

Bite marks are a clear example of crush injuries (Fig. 101). Each tooth compresses the skin and underlying tissues, crushing them. When fresh, an individual bruise is seen under each tooth, and an impression of the tooth is seen in the skin, possibly with a break in the skin's surface. Human bites can be distinguished from other mammal bites by the relative width of the arch in proportion to its depth, and by the absence of long sharp canines. The upper adult arch can be distinguished from the lower because all lower incisors are the same width, while the upper central are wider than the upper lateral incisors. Many measurements have been made on human dentition, but the most reliable measurement for distinguishing adult from immature dentition is the upper inter-canine distance, which is less than 3 cm in immature dentition, and wider in the adult.

Another crush type injury is a pinch (Fig. 102). The appearance of two ovate bruises across a central clearing suggests pinching. The size and shape of the bruises depends on whether the pinching part was a knuckle or finger tip. When fingernails are used, a laceration or abrasion may lie at the outer edge of one or both of the paired bruises.

Chafing or stretching is the cause of bruising in ligature marks (Fig. 103). These marks appear as circumferential, or near-circumferential injuries, usually at the wrists or ankles. Skip areas may occur under knots, or where the ligature is lifted off the skin by connection to the opposite extremity or the object to which the victim was tied. ➡

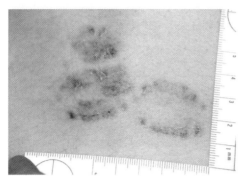

Fig. 101 Multiple bite marks on a child's back.

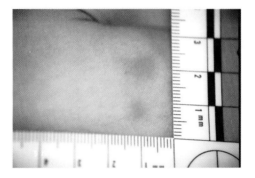

Fig. 102 Pinch marks on a child's arm.

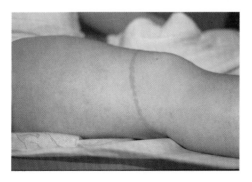

Fig. 103 Encircling ligature mark on a child's thigh.

Injuries need not have an identifiable shape in order to be suspicious. A distinct shape, which cannot be identified, but recurs, is suggestive of some repeated human activity (Fig. 104). Studies in Great Britain and the USA have shown that infants who cannot pull up and walk along furniture seldom have any bruises, and very rarely more than two. Accidental bruises in young children often involve the shins, thighs, forehead and scalp, but very rarely the face and buttocks. Excess bruising, facial bruising and buttock bruising in infants and toddlers can indicate abuse.

The ears and buttocks have demonstrated special, recognizable, patterns of bruising. During paddling, bruises may develop parallel to the gluteal cleft (Fig.105). These injuries are thought to arise as the buttocks come rapidly together, forming an abrupt angle where the cleft meets the impacting object. Blows to the ears can result in petechiae and small bruises within the curves and along the superior edge of the pinna (Fig. 106). These injuries may be hidden in hair or shadow and missed if not looked for. Both these forms of injury were originally described in abused children, and are rarely seen in other situations.

Many texts have suggested that the colour of a bruise can be used to determine its age. Recent data shows this to be untrue, and supports the following conclusions on bruise coloration.

- red may be visible at any time;
- yellow may appear 18–24 hours after injury;
- two bruises of the same age may be different colours.

The progression of colour change over time is useful for distinguishing bruises from other findings, and fresh injuries from much older ones, but exact bruise dating is strongly discouraged. ➡

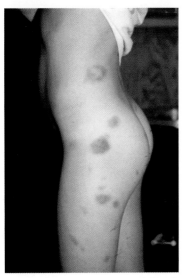

Fig. 104 Multiple patterned bruises inflicted on a child with Von Willebrand's disease.

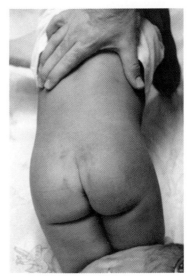

Fig. 105 Paddling bruises parallel to the gluteal cleft.

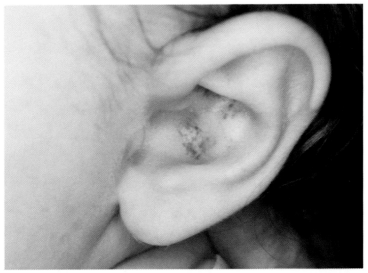

Fig. 106 Petechiae within the recesses of a child's ear.

The most common conditions confused with abusive bruises are disorders of coagulation and dermatological conditions that may simulate bruising.

Coagulation disorders may be permanent or temporary. The classic haemophilias can result in bruising at a young age, numerous vigorous bruises, or patterned bruises from common household trauma but a history of haemarthrosis, or family history of the disorder is often present, making misdiagnosis less likely. Von Willebrand's disease, however, demonstrates significant variability in penetrance, so that affected parents may be unaware that they have the disorder. Patterned bruises in these patients have the same significance as to causation, but less implied force than the same bruise in a normal child (Fig. 104).

Idiopathic, or immune thrombocytopenic purpura is a relatively common, temporary clotting disorder (Fig. 107). The sudden appearance of multiple bruises on a young child may raise concerns for child abuse. Though not a disorder of coagulation, Henoch Schoenlein, or anaphylactoid purpura, also presents with sudden onset of bruising, most typically of the lower extremities and buttocks. Studies of coagulation and a blood count are called for whenever evaluating bruising for suspicious cause.

Both pigmentary and vascular lesions have been mistaken for bruising (Figs 108 and 109). Many people are unfamiliar with mongolian, or slate-grey spots (Fig. 110), and when they first see these blue-black blotches on the sacrum and buttocks may believe them to be bruises from spanking. The ability of vascular lesions to blanch can immediately distinguish them from bruising. Follow-up examination, demonstrating the lack of expected resolution with time, will distinguish pigmentary lesions from bruises. ➡

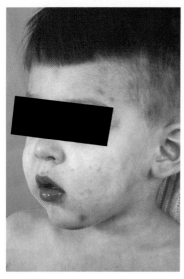

Fig. 107 Multiple facial bruises in a child with immune thrombocytopenic purpura.

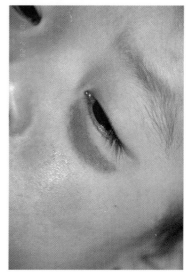

Fig. 108 Congenital naevus simulating a black eye.

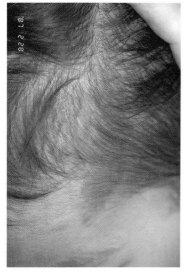

Fig. 109 Port wine stain on the head of the patient shown in Fig. 108.

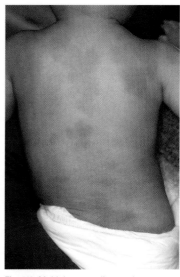

Fig. 110 Multiple mongolian or slate-grey spots.

Burns

Some authors have suggested that there is no burn pattern which is specific for abuse, that it is the inconsistency between the given history and either the pattern of the burn or the child's developmental abilities which most commonly indicates undisclosed inflicted injury. Certain patterns, however, are so characteristic of abuse as to be consistent with little else, and research has demonstrated a close association between other burn findings and inflicted injury.

Patterned injuries

In much of the European literature, dry contact burns are the most common form of abusive burning. In children under 4 years old, where abusive burns tend to occur, 50% of contact burns are inflicted. Accidental contact burns tend to occur when a running or falling child brushes against a hot object, or a hot object falls, striking a child. The motion of the patient or hot object produces irregular margins which give evidence of this movement. In contrast, abusers inflict burns by pressing hot objects into the skin of restrained children. The result is a sharp outline of the object. These burns may have a readily recognizable shape, such as a steam iron, or metal grate (Fig. 111). The classic cigarette burn is a sharply demarcated 8 mm circular crater surrounded by a raised rolled edge (Fig. 112). Shallower burns with a distinct 8mm circle are also likely to be from cigarettes. Burning is a torturous activity, and may therefore be a repetitive activity. When multiple distinct burns are seen, especially with a recognizable pattern, inflicted injury is certain (Fig. 113).

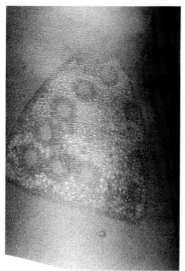

Fig. 111 Burn on the chest, inflicted with a steam iron.

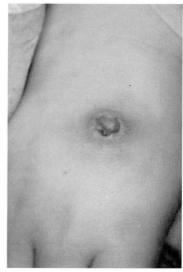

Fig. 112 Burn on the hand, inflicted with a cigarette.

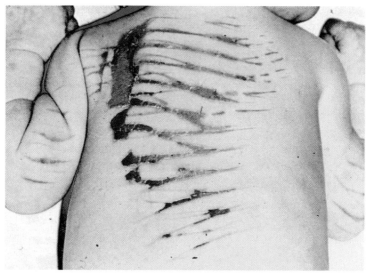

Fig. 113 Multiple overlapping burns, inflicted with a heated metal grate.

In most American studies, hot water scalds are the most common form of abusive burn injury, although they are not abusive as often as contact burns: 10–20% of paediatric scald burns necessitating hospitalization are caused by abuse. Usually abuse is diagnosed because the given history fails to match the burn pattern or the developmental abilities of the child. The classic tub immersion pattern, however, is readily recognized and highly associated with abuse (Figs 114 and 115). In these cases confluent and uniform burning of the lower body occurs, but may spare flexural creases, the buttocks, the knees and toes. While the pattern may at first appear complex, positioning the child in the right manner reveals that the superior margin of the burn forms a straight line, which is parallel to the ground when the child is reclining or sitting. This sort of margin is also referred to as a 'high-tide line' and marks the upper limit of the hot water during immersion. Splash marks are minimal or absent in most cases. The depth of the burn, sharp margins, and the absence of splash marks suggests that these children are rapidly dipped into very hot water, at least 60°C.

Other findings have been associated with inflicted burn injuries. Burns that show evidence of delayed care seeking, in the form of infection or healing, symmetrical or 'mirror image' burns and the presence of associated injuries all occur much more frequently in child abuse (Figs 115 and 116). Initial suspicion and careful evaluation may be necessary, as close examination of the ears, mouth, or genitals, and skeletal radiography may be necessary to find the additional injuries. These cases fall under the category of the 'battered child syndrome', defined by the presence of multiple distinct injuries, without adequate explanation. This syndrome has been recognized since 1962 as an indication of inflicted injury. ➡

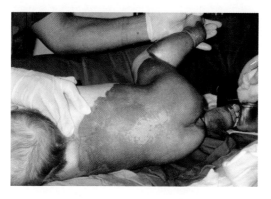

Fig. 114 Tub immersion burn, showing high tide line.

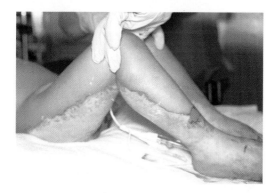

Fig. 115 Tub immersion burn with evidence of healing, and high tide line.

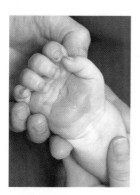 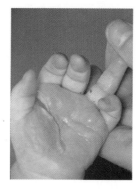

Fig. 116 Symmetrical burning of both palms.

Of all the conditions mistaken for abuse, bullous impetigo creates the most confusion (Fig. 117). This condition may form multiple sharply marginated circular ulcers, which have been mistaken for cigarette burns. The superficial nature of the ulcers, the presence of honey-coloured crusts, and spread in the absence of treatment will distinguish impetigo.

Skeletal injury

After cutaneous injuries, skeletal injury is the next most commonly identified evidence of child abuse. Certain fractures are commonly and exclusively associated with abuse, making them a form of patterned injury. Rib fractures in infants are strongly associated with abuse, and posterior rib fractures, adjacent to the lateral process of the spine, occur almost exclusively in inflicted injury (Fig. 118). Computerized tomography, histopathology, and animal experimentation have all suggested that these fractures are formed when the chest is grabbed and squeezed. The posterior rib is levered over the transverse process of the spine, stressing and cracking the internal cortex. This fracture is initially a very subtle finding, becoming more apparent as it heals and forms callous.

Fracture at the ends of long bones, known as the 'classical metaphyseal lesion', has been considered the skeletal injury most pathognomonic for child abuse (Fig. 119). These injuries were initially thought to be avulsion injuries at the insertion of articular ligaments. Hisopathology has shown the small radiologically evident injury to be caused by a larger break through the physeal cartilage. The epiphyseal end carries with it a ring of calcified tissue that may appear as an arc or 'bucket handle', or a 'corner chip' at the ends of the bone. Like rib fractures, these injuries may initially be subtle; unlike rib fractures they do not reliably heal with visible callous formation. ➡

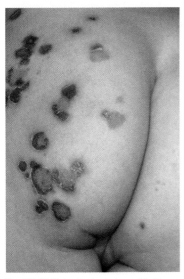

Fig. 117 Multiple circular lesions of bullous impetigo.

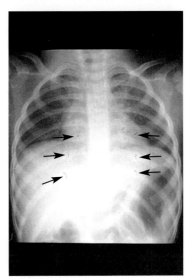

Fig. 118 Chest radiograph showing multiple posterior rib fractures (arrow).

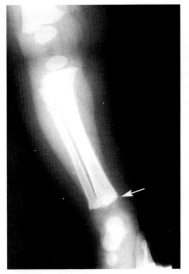

Fig. 119 (a) Classic metaphyseal lesion, seen as a 'bucket handle' at the end of the tibia (arrow).

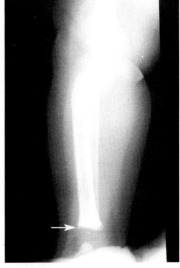

Fig. 119 (b) Lateral view of the same fracture, showing the 'corner chip' configuration (arrow).

Some studies suggest that most inflicted skeletal injuries, like accidental injuries, involve diaphyseal fractures of long bones. The child's age is often the first thing that raises the likelihood of abuse in these children. 80% of abusive fractures occur in children under 18 months, while only 2% of accidental fractures occur in this age range. Up to 50% of fractures in children under 1 year are due to inflicted injury. Inconsistent explanatory history, evidence of delayed care in the form of fracture healing (Fig. 120) and additional unexplained injuries give further evidence supporting abuse. Because long bone fractures may be dated by their state of healing, the presence of new fractures on old may be all that is needed to diagnose the 'battered child syndrome' and child abuse (Fig. 121).

A variety of conditions may cause skeletal findings simulating fracture or genuine fracture through bone fragility. The most frequently discussed of these is osteogenesis imperfecta, a congenital disorder of collagen synthesis which results in brittle bones (Fig. 122). The presence of blue sclerae, short stature, congenital fractures, brittle teeth, pre-senile hearing loss, osteopenia on radiograph or multiple wormian bones of the skull in the child, or the family history, will usually identify children with this condition. Children who were born prematurely, and received parenteral nutrition, who are bedridden with neurodevelopmental handicaps or who have chronic renal failure may develop metabolic bone disease and fragility. Vitamin D-deficient rickets, Menke's kinky hair syndrome, and congenital syphilis all produce skeletal changes that have been mistaken for trauma. In the first two conditions, changes occur at the metaphyses of long bones, and must be distinguished from the 'classical metaphyseal lesion'.➡

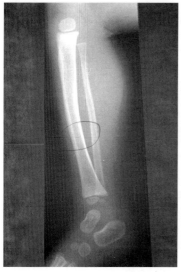

Fig. 120 (a) Fresh transverse fracture of the tibia with bowing deformity of the fibula.

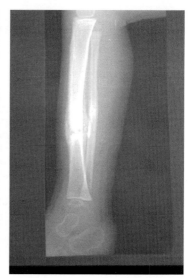

Fig. 120 (b) Same fracture 4 weeks later, with periosteal new bone and widening of the fracture line.

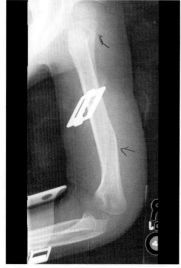

Fig. 121 Multiple fractures of the humerus in different stages of healing.

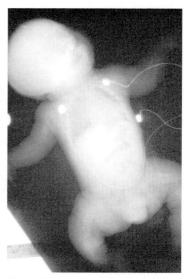

Fig. 122 Whole-body radiograph of a child with severe osteogenesis imperfecta.

Internal injuries

Many serious internal injuries have resulted from
child abuse. Whenever internal injuries occur in
young children without explanation, or explained
by trivial household trauma, child abuse should be
suspected. Head injury is the most important
example of this group because it is the most
common, and causes the most deaths and
disability. Serious head injuries may occur without
any external evidence of trauma, a situation which
led to the original description of the 'shaken baby'
syndrome. Whenever a subdural haematoma or
subarachnoid haematoma occurs with associated
brain injury, but without historical evidence of
serious trauma, abusive head injury should be
suspected (Fig. 123). Many of these children will
have skeletal injuries, as originally described in the
'shaken baby' syndrome, and most will have retinal
haemorrhages, a finding itself strongly associated
with child abuse (Fig. 124). Many also have external
injuries and evidence of impact to the head. Some
authors have suggested that shaking alone is
not enough to cause serious head injuries. Unless
specific evidence of shaking is present, the term
abusive head trauma is suggested to describe
these patients.

Many other forms of visceral injury have been
described as a result of child abuse. Pharyngeal
laceration, rupture or haematoma of the duodenum
and proximal jejunum (Fig. 125) and lacerations
and haematomas of the pancreas and left lobe of
the liver are particularly common results of inflicted
injury. These cases are identified by an inconsistent
history that lacks explanatory trauma and evidence
of delay in care seeking. While this form of abusive
injury is relatively rare, it has the highest mortality
rate of all forms of abuse, making it the second
most common cause of abuse death.

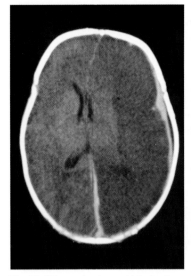

Fig. 123 CT scan showing multiple density subdural haematoma, and ipsilateral brain oedema with mass effect.

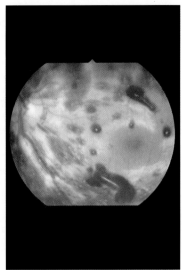

Fig. 124 Extensive retinal haemorrhages involving multiple levels of the retina.

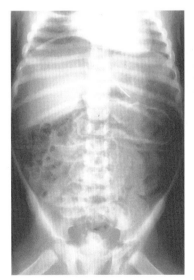

Fig. 125 (a) Plain film of the abdomen with pneumoperitoneum.

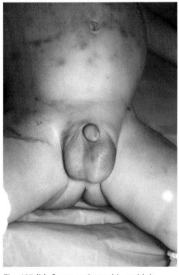

Fig. 125 (b) Same patient with multiple abdominal and scrotal haematomas.

Sexual abuse

While it is often difficult for medical providers to acknowledge the possibility of physical abuse, it may be even harder to face the reality of sexual abuse. Most cases are recognized through adult suspicions, sexualized child behaviours, and statements made by the child. Delayed presentation, non-intrusive abuse practices, and remarkable healing make physical evidence of trauma the exception rather than the rule. Limited knowledge of genital anatomy, unfamiliarity with special examination techniques, and public controversy over this diagnosis may further reduce a provider's sensitivity to the findings that do exist.

Examination techniques

Simply placing a girl in the prone position and spreading her legs typically results in a view of the labia majora, perhaps with some labia minora protruding. Some labial separation is needed to see the internal genital structures. To reliably open the hymenal orifice and define the anatomy of this important structure, special techniques are necessary. Grasping the labia majora and drawing them out, away from the body, will elongate the vestibule, and dilate the vaginal canal, causing the hymen to open and spread out (Fig. 126). Further dilation of the vaginal canal can be gained by putting the child in the prone 'knee chest' position, in which the hymen will tend to fall forward and elongate, affording an excellent view of its anatomy (Figs 127 and 128). In some cases the hymen will stick to itself or to adjacent structures. The application of warm water or normal saline can release the surface tension, allowing the hymen to drape or float so that it can be fully defined. ➡

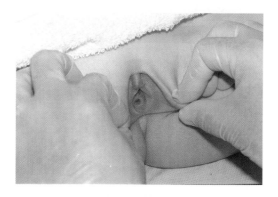

Fig. 126 Labial traction is used to separate the edges of the hymen.

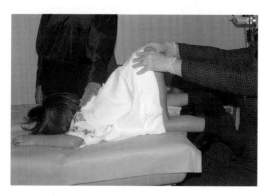

Fig. 127 Child in the prone 'knee chest' position.

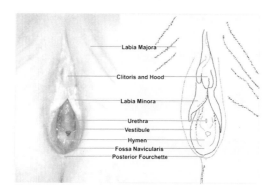

Labia Majora
Clitoris and Hood
Labia Minora
Urethra
Vestibule
Hymen
Fossa Navicularis
Posterior Fourchette

Fig. 128 Important genital structures.

Acute female genital injuries

While physical findings are identified in only approximately 25% of all cases, the likelihood rises to 50% with report of bleeding, and to 69% if the examination is carried out within 72 hours. Some acute findings are minor, such as genital haematomas, submucosal haemorrhage, petechiae, abrasions, oedema, or simple erythema (Fig. 129). These injuries may disappear in a matter of days, and follow-up examination is essential to be sure they disappear as expected. At times capillary loops or haemangiomas have been mistaken for petechiae or haematomas.

Blunt trauma from attempted intromission may result in lacerations. These may be minor, involving only the edge of the hymen, with limited bleeding (Fig. 130). Such injuries will also heal rapidly, and may leave only a small change in the hymenal contour or a smooth but subtly narrower hymen. The most violent of assaults may result in lacerations through the hymen and extending into the fossa navicularis, vaginal wall or posterior fourchette (Fig. 131). Rarely these lesions have perforated into the peritoneum, causing serious illness. In most cases, even this severe form of sexual trauma will heal quite rapidly without treatment. Resolution of oedema, and the formation of granulation tissue on denuded subcutaneous tissues, can be seen within 24 hours (Fig. 131). Defects will fill in and epithelium regenerate to resolve deep lacerations within 1–2 weeks. The vagina, fossa and fourchette will probably heal without a trace; permanent scarring being unusual. While a defect is likely to persist in the hymen, in the form of a transection, the base of the hymen may appear to regenerate, leaving a deep, but incomplete cleft. Whether a cleft or transection is formed, this irregularity will smooth out and lose its jagged appearance over the weeks to months that follow. ➡

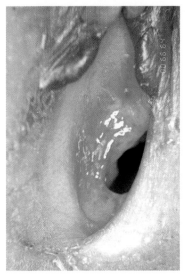

Fig. 129 Submucosal haemorrhage of the hymen and adjacent vestibule.

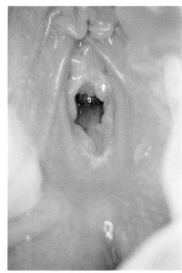

Fig. 130 Small fresh partial-thickness tear of the hymen at 3 o'clock.

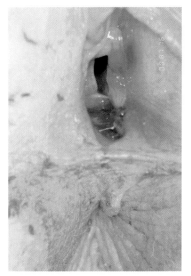

Fig. 131 (a) Acute laceration through the posterior hymen, extending into the fossa navicularis and posterior vaginal wall.

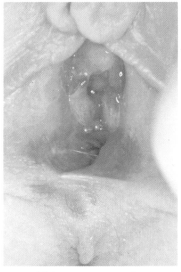

Fig. 131 (b) Same child 36 hours later. Granulation tissue may be seen in the laceration.

Healed female genital injuries

Most child sexual abuse progresses secretly over time by coercion and accommodation. The disclosure or discovery of the abuse is often delayed and initially unconvincing. Given this situation most injuries have healed by the time the child is brought for examination. The focus of the delayed exam becomes the hymen, the one tissue which is likely to show evidence of abuse that occurred months or even years earlier.

The hymenal finding most clearly indicative of past sexual trauma is the transection, also known as the complete cleft (Fig. 132). A break in the inferior hymen extending completely through to the vaginal wall has never been described in a non-abused child. Longitudinal studies of lacerations sustained during acute sexual assault have documented the subsequent development of transection. Only accidental penetrating genital injury presents an alternative diagnostic possibility in these cases.

Notches on the posterior hymen, also called concavities or clefts, are often cited as evidence of sexual trauma (Fig. 133). This finding has also been documented as arising from acute traumatic laceration. Normal mounds, folds or fimbriation at times create confusion (Fig. 134), particularly in the neonate or adolescent, when the hymen is typically wide and redundant. The relative depth of the notch is often used to resolve this issue. Determining this proportion is complicated by difficulties in identifying the true base of the hymen.

General hymenal narrowing is the most controversial hymenal finding (Fig. 135). Hymenal narrowing has also been seen to develop in the wake of acute injury. Given the aforementioned difficulty in identifying the hymenal base, it is sometimes difficult to determine when a hymen is too narrow to be normal.

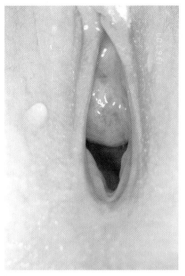

Fig. 132 Transection of the hymen at the 6 o'clock position.

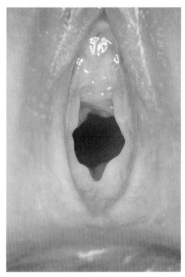

Fig. 133 Deep but incomplete cleft at the 6 o'clock position.

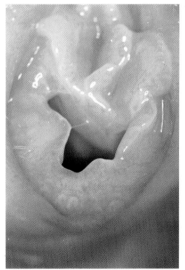

Fig. 134 Adolescent hymen with irregular edge.

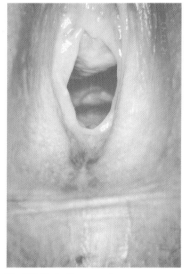

Fig. 135 Markedly narrow hymen.

Anal injuries

Acute injuries found after anal penetration include bruising of perianal tissue and lacerations (Fig. 136). Multiple irregular lacerations are clear evidence of sexual assault, but subtle, non-specific injuries such as superficial abrasions and small perianal fissures may be more common. In cases with severe trauma, a period of anal laxity or flaccidity may occur. Anal injuries, like injuries of the posterior fourchette and fossa navicularis, usually heal rapidly and completely, leaving no scar or trace.

Almost all findings in the delayed anal examination are controversial. The presence of anal dilation, once believed to be evidence of recurrent anal penetration, is inconsistently cited today, and then only when there is immediate dilation greater than 2 cm in the absence of rectal stool (Fig. 137). Tags off the midline, and areas of venous engorgement, may cause concern for past trauma, but are seldom taken as clear evidence of sexual abuse. The presence of scarring is felt to be clear evidence of past injury, but is so seldom seen, that serious scrutiny is necessary before identifying any finding as a scar.

Male genital injuries

Discussion of male sexual abuse usually focuses on the anal findings discussed above. Male genital injuries are more commonly seen in child physical abuse, due to corporal punishment or ligation to prevent urination. Haematomas, lacerations and abrasions may be found (Fig. 138) and prolonged ligation may produce oedema or ischaemia. The latter condition must be distinguished from a hair or thread tourniquet, a known accidental injury. Vigorous suction during oral copulation may produce petechiae on the head of the penis (Fig. 139), and at times tooth marks may be seen, but penile injuries following sexual abuse are rare.

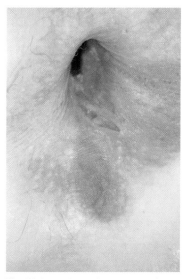

Fig. 136 Laceration and haematoma of the anus, with mild laxity.

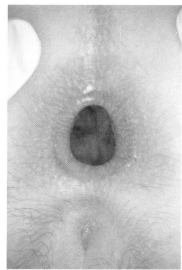

Fig. 137 Markedly dilated anus with no stool present.

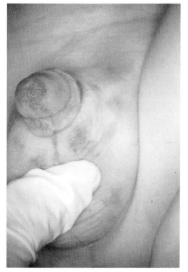

Fig. 138 Penile and scrotal haematomas.

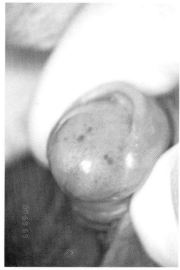

Fig. 139 Petechiae of the glans penis following oral copulation.

Variation and non-specific conditions

Conditions mistaken for abuse

Several findings were first identified in abused children and believed to be post-traumatic, until they were found in girls selected for non-abuse. Mounds on the edge of the hymen, bands of tissue between the hymen and the lateral vestibule, and intravaginal ridges that connect to the hymen are now known to be normal structures. Many variants mistaken for acute or healing trauma occur along the midline. Linea vestibularis is a midline avascular streak in the posterior fourchette and fossa navicularis (Fig. 140). A depressed groove, found in this area during puberty, is still felt by some to be due to trauma. Smooth depressed areas, known as diastasis ani, occur on the anterior or posterior perianal midline. A mucosa-lined depression called perineal groove, or failure of midline fusion, may extend along the raphe from the anus toward the posterior fourchette (Fig. 141). These findings are all found in non-abused children, and are not signs of abuse.

Medical conditions have also resulted in unfounded concern for sexual abuse. Non-specific and streptococcal vaginitis cause genital erythema and discharge, which may be mistaken for trauma or a sexually transmitted disease. Urethral prolapse produces a large bleeding mass, which may appear to be an injured hymen (Fig. 142). Lichen sclerosis et atrophicus is a condition that produces sharply demarcated, thin, hypopigmented and fragile skin surrounding the anus and genitals (Fig. 143). Itching due to associated pruritis may result in haemorrhage and abrasion, which can be mistaken for inflicted injury. Most accidental trauma produces injuries of the labia majora, labia minora and, rarely, the fourchette. Accidental hymenal trauma is uncommon, and presents with dramatic explanatory history. As in all forms of abuse, matching the history to the findings is crucial in determining whether a child was abused and by whom.

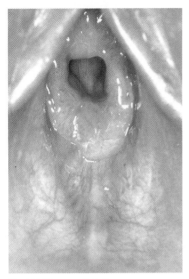

Fig. 140 Linea vestibularis.

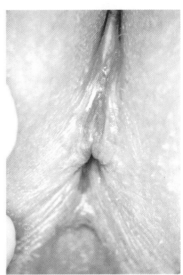

Fig. 141 Failure of midline fusion anterior to the anus with diastasis ani posteriorly.

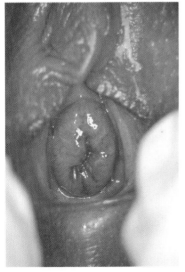

Fig. 142 Marked urethral prolapse.

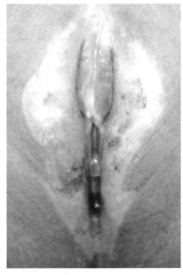

Fig. 143 Lichen sclerosis et atrophicus with abrasion and haematoma of the labia majora.

Deliberate self-harm may have two outcomes –
death or survival. Chapter 5 refers to typical
patterns of self-inflicted harm in the living. The
diagnosis of death by an individual's own hand is
of great medicolegal importance, with specific
relevance to insurance claims, coroner's decisions
and pursuance of criminal proceedings: homicides
may be disguised as suicides; a suicide may be
disguised as an accident for insurance purposes;
accidents may appear as suicide. Thus, the
investigation and assessment of all sudden and
unexpected deaths is of major significance in all
jurisdictions.

Methods of suicide are similar on a global basis,
although there is individual variation in the specific
means taken depending on the local availability of
methods. In all investigations of suspected suicides,
the previous medical and social history of an
individual may give specific indications as to the
potential for self-harm and whether a death may
have been a failed 'cry for help' or a clear intention
to end life. In some jurisdictions (e.g. England and
Wales) a criminal standard of proof (i.e. beyond
reasonable doubt) is used to determine suicide for
statutory purposes.

Suicide may be undertaken in many ways – in
some cases, methods may be combined (e.g. alcohol,
drugs and car exhausts). The most commonly seen
methods include:

- hanging/suspension (Figs 144 and 145);
- drug overdoses/poisoning;
- firearms (Fig. 146);
- carbon monoxide (car exhaust fumes);
- asphyxia;
- electrocution;
- fire/self-immolation;
- jumping from heights;
- railways (i.e. lying on a railway line, usually with
  the neck on the rail);
- motor vehicles; and
- sharp blades (stabbing, incising).

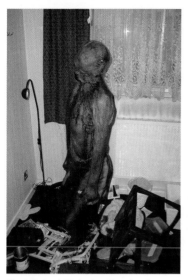

Fig. 144 A suicide by hanging showing decomposition.

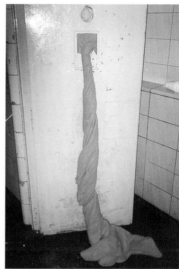

Fig. 145 Blanket used for attempted suicide by hanging in a prison cell.

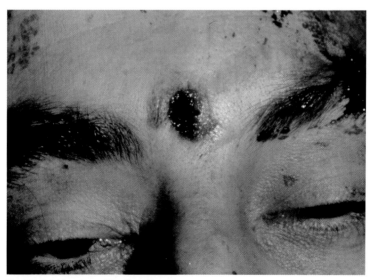

Fig. 146 Suicide using a .22 calibre rifle.

9 Motor vehicle accidents

Incidents involving motor vehicles often result in medicolegal issues that require medical input. The pathologist will be the principal doctor involved with fatalities. Clinicians will treat living casualties but may also be required to examine fatalities. When doing so, the medicolegal issues should never be forgotten. A history of the events and a thorough examination of the patient or body and documentation of the findings are essential. An examination should be made of the clothing worn by the victim and the collection of any foreign bodies or substance within clothing, wounds, etc., as these may assist in the identification of the vehicles involved, particularly in 'hit and run' cases.

Pedestrians

Injuries sustained by pedestrians can result from three sources:

- direct impact with the vehicle;
- striking the ground or other objects;
- other vehicles either running over or striking the victim.

Motor vehicles

The nature of the injuries sustained by the occupants of motor vehicles will depend upon the circumstances of the accident. Often it is important to determine who was driving the vehicle, and the presence of seat belt markings can assist. Most accidents are frontal impacts, which result in injuries due to rapid deceleration. Occupants of the front seats tend to sustain the more severe injuries, which may include:

- forehead injuries due to hitting the windscreen and or side pillars;
- chest injuries from the steering column;
- knee injuries from hitting the dashboard;
- lower limb injuries from transmitted stress (Fig. 147).

If seat belts are not worn the injuries may be more extensive and the victim may be projected out of the vehicle. It is important to note that the extent of injuries sustained cannot be directly correlated with the damage sustained by the vehicle, as illustrated in Fig. 148. Here, a pedestrian, after being hit by the vehicle, was thrown onto the bonnet and then the road, walked from the scene with minor bruising only.

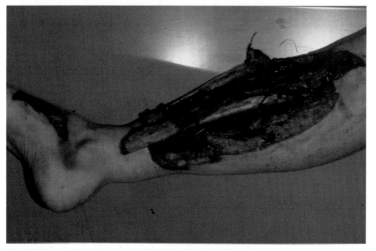

Fig. 147 Fractured leg among other injuries sustained after a head-on collision.

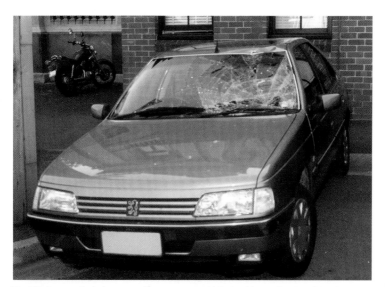

Fig. 148 Damaged windscreen and bonnet on a vehicle that hit a pedestrian allegedly at 60 kph.

Ethanol (alcohol) is an important aspect of forensic medicine, given its association with crimes and motor vehicle accidents. As it is common for doctors to be called upon to assess an alcohol-affected person or give evidence in court regarding its effects and involvement in various crimes and driving incidents, an understanding of alcohol is essential. Doctors and nurses may also be required to collect blood samples using approved kits (Fig. 149) for evidentiary use.

Alcohol is a central nervous system depressant and its acute effects range from sobriety through euphoria and excitement to drunkenness, stupor, coma and death. After ingestion, alcohol is absorbed into the bloodstream and distributed throughout the body. Most alcohol is metabolized by the liver and excreted. The rate of absorption, metabolism and excretion varies due to a number of factors, including:

- the presence or absence of food in the stomach (a full stomach may reduce the peak alcohol concentration by up to 20%);
- the rate of drinking;
- the nature and alcoholic strength of the beverage;
- the sex and physical build of the drinker;
- the presence of any residual alcohol in the circulation;
- the presence of drugs that may increase (e.g. metoclopramide, erythromycin, cisapride) or decrease (e.g. atropine, tricyclic antidepressants, opiates) the rate of gastric emptying;
- the emotional state of the drinker;
- the habituation to alcohol of the drinker.

The peak level of alcohol in the bloodstream is attained 30–120 minutes (usually about 45) after drinking. Following absorption, there is an elimination phase during which the alcohol is metabolized and excreted from the body. It is during this elimination phase that blood alcohol concentrations can be estimated and 'read-backs' estimated for court purposes (Fig. 150).

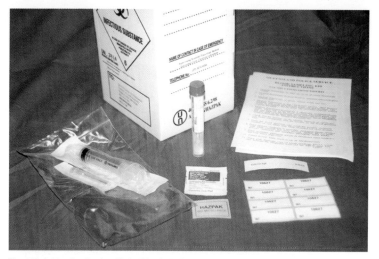

Fig. 149 A blood collection kit for blood alcohol estimation. These vary between jurisdictions.

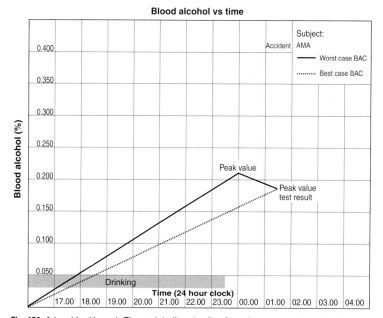

Fig. 150 A 'read-back' graph. The straight lines leading from time zero to the peak values should be a curve and, therefore, this does not represent the actual blood alcohol concentrations during that period.

Substance use and misuse are major problems in modern society. Drug use, especially when associated with drug dependence, is often associated with criminal activity. This may be related to the direct effect of the drug (driving or committing a criminal offence whilst under the influence), the economic effects (offences committed for the purpose of acquiring money to buy the drug) and the criminal links related to selling, manufacturing and distributing the drug (Fig. 151).

Definition

A drug of abuse is any substance, taken through any route of administration that alters the mood, the level of perception, or brain functioning and used in a way that differs from approved medical practice.

Drug dependence occurs when the user feels he or she needs the drug to function optimally (psychological dependence) or the body has adapted physiologically to chronic use of the drug and develops physical symptoms when the drug is withdrawn (physical dependence).

Illicit drugs are those which are acquired and used in an illegal or socially unacceptable fashion.

Two important aspects of physical dependence are:

- development of *tolerance* to the drug, with the need for higher doses to achieve the same effect
- development of a *withdrawal* or abstinence syndrome with a wide variety of symptoms.

Effects

Doctors need to be able to recognize the effects of the commonly used illicit drugs. This involves understanding and recognizing the direct effects of the commonly used drugs, the symptoms and signs of drug dependence, withdrawal and the long-term physical and psychological effects of illicit drug use. Associated medical and psychiatric conditions related to illicit drug use (especially intravenous drug use) include:

- damage to superficial veins (Figs 152 and 153);
- deep vein thrombosis and pulmonary embolus; ➡

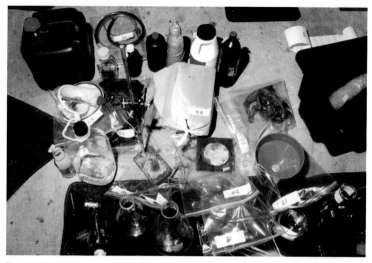

Fig. 151 Illicit amphetamine laboratory.

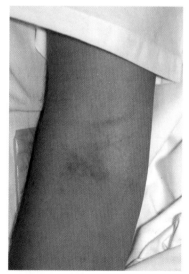

Fig. 152 IV track sites in the antecubital fossa.

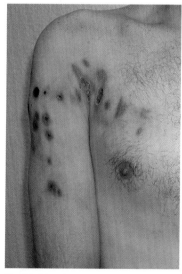

Fig. 153 IV marks on the upper arm and chest.

- acute and subacute bacterial endocarditis;
- sepsis/septicaemia;
- dental caries and periodontal disease;
- HIV and hepatitis especially hepatitis B and C;
- psychiatric conditions including psychosis and depression;
- suicide or sudden accidental death from overdose.

Once the problem has been identified in a patient, a treatment programme needs to be considered. This involves education relating to minimization of harm, withdrawal from the drug and removal of the patient from the drug-using environment, and long-term medical and psychosocial support.

Common illicit drugs (Fig. 154) include narcotic analgesics, benzodiazepines, stimulants, cannabis and hallucinogens.

Narcotic analgesics

Opiates (drugs derived from opium) and opioids (synthetic narcotics) are useful and medically important drugs as they have effective analgesic properties. However, there is a high potential for misuse especially with the major opiates (heroin, morphine and codeine) and opioids such as methadone.

Opiates may be taken orally, by injection (subcutaneous, intramuscular or intravenous) by sniffing or inhalation or by dermal patches. Heroin is the most common illicit opiate and is commonly taken by intravenous injection (Fig. 155) or inhalation. Heroin is a depressant of the central nervous and cardiac systems. The predominant physical effects of heroin or morphine include pinpoint pupils, respiratory depression, bradycardia, suppression of the cough reflex, constipation, nausea, vomiting and drowsiness. Psychological effects include analgesia, reduction of anxiety, inability to concentrate with some clouding of mental functioning and euphoria and a feeling of contentment. Similar effects are noted with methadone and, to a lesser extent, with codeine. Tolerance, physical and psychological dependence occur.

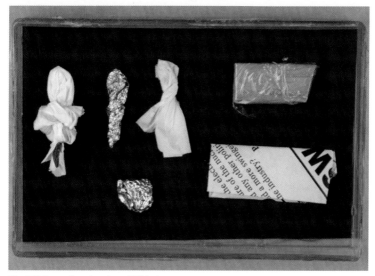

Fig. 154 Examples of packaged illicit drugs.

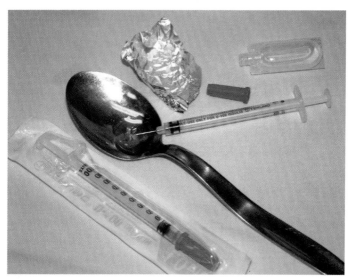

Fig. 155 Intravenous drug paraphernalia.

The severity of the physical dependence will depend on the opiate (Fig. 156), dose, duration of use, and clinical aspects such as the presence of severe pain or sepsis (Fig. 157). Psychological dependence may persist long after physical withdrawal.

Withdrawal or abstinence syndrome occurs after stopping the drug. The onset, severity and duration will depend on the type of drug used and to a lesser extent on the user's expectations. Heroin withdrawal occurs within a few hours of the last dose and reaches a peak at 2–4 days. The symptoms then settle rapidly. Methadone has a much longer half-life, with symptoms developing at 24 hours and persisting for 10–14 days.

Withdrawal

Symptoms of withdrawal include:

- goose bumps and feeling hot and cold;
- yawning;
- anorexia, abdominal cramps, nausea, vomiting and diarrhoea;
- generalized aches and pains;
- tremor and weakness;
- insomnia.

Signs of withdrawal include:

- dilated pupils;
- sweating and piloerection;
- rhinorrhoea and lacrimation;
- tachycardia and elevated blood pressure;
- restlessness and anxiety.

Withdrawal may be assisted medically by substitution of another opiate such as methadone or buprenorphine.

Symptomatic treatment

Symptomatic treatment may include:

- *diazepam* – up to 40 mg per day for anxiety;
- *Lomotil* (*diphenoxylate and atropine*) for diarrhoea;
- *metaclopramide* 10 mg three times a day or *promethazine* 25 mg at night for nausea;
- *buscopan* 10 mg three times a day for bowel spasm;
- *paracetamol* 1000 mg or *ibuprofen* 400 mg for aches and pains;
- *clonidine* or *lofexidine* – alpha-adrenergic drugs, which are effective but should be used with care due to their hypotensive and sedating effects. ➡

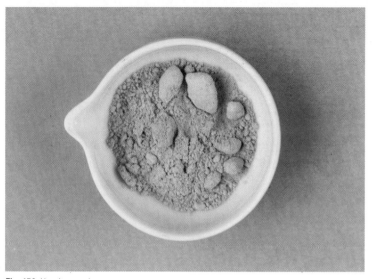

Fig. 156 Heroin powder.

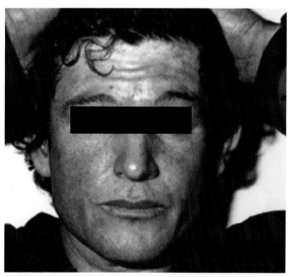

Fig. 157 Facial staphylococcal sepsis from intravenous drug use.

Relapse from treatment is common without continuing intensive psychosocial support, which may be needed long term.

Benzodiazepines

Benzodiazepines (Fig. 158) are central nervous system depressants and are used as sedatives, anxiolytics and hypnotics. They may also be used to reduce muscle spasm and in the treatment of epilepsy. The group includes diazepam and clonazepam (long acting), temazepam, nitrazepam (medium acting) and flunitrazepam (short acting).

Tolerance, physical and psychological dependence occur rapidly and there is cross-tolerance with alcohol and barbiturate hypnotics.

Poly-drug use involving opiates, alcohol, cannabis and benzodiazepines is common.

Physical effects

Physical effects of acute intoxication include dizziness, sedation (Fig. 159), uncoordination, slurred speech, difficulty in concentrating, low blood pressure and respiratory depression. Death is uncommon unless the drug has been used with other central nervous system depressants. A person's ability to safely operate a motor vehicle or machinery may be impaired.

Psychological effects include relief of anxiety and promotion of relaxation. Memory impairment and emotional lability may occur and there may be paradoxical behaviour with aggression or other inappropriate reactions to situations.

A withdrawal syndrome may occur, with anxiety, sweating, insomnia and headache. Seizures and psychosis may also be associated with withdrawal, especially if high doses of benzodiazepines have been used for extended periods. Withdrawal is managed by replacement with diazepam and reduction over a period of time (up to several months). ➡

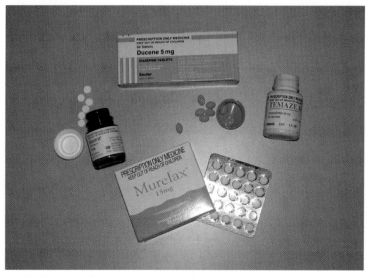

Fig. 158 Some benzodiazepines pharmaceutically available.

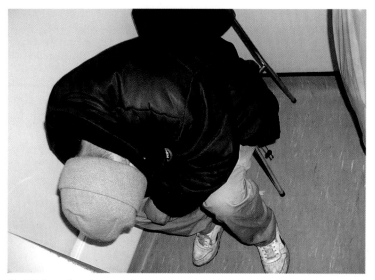

Fig. 159 Benzodiazepine user asleep.

Cannabis

After alcohol, nicotine and caffeine, cannabis is the most widely used recreational drug. Cannabis, also known as marijuana, pot, hashish, charas, bhang and ganga, is the most commonly used illicit drug in the world.

Cannabis is derived from the plant *Cannabis sativa* (Fig. 160). It has several active chemical components, the most active of which is Δ-9-tetrahydrocannabinol (THC). *Cannabis sativa* grows readily in warm climates. Plants grown hydroponically under artificial lights have a higher concentration of THC than plants grown naturally. The highest concentration of THC is found in the flower heads (Fig. 161), with lower levels in the leaves and the lowest in the stem.

Cannabis may be smoked or ingested (Fig. 162). THC is absorbed very quickly from the lungs. After smoking, the plasma level peaks at 10 minutes and intoxication lasts 2–3 hours. When ingested orally, the effect lasts longer. The drug disappears from the blood rapidly, passing into the tissues with special affinity for fatty tissues. The half-life of THC is 7 days. A single dose may take 30 days for complete elimination and chronic use may lead to an accumulation of THC and metabolites in the body.

Effects

These include euphoria, feeling of relaxation, sleepiness, inability to keep track of time, hunger, decreased social interaction, short-term memory loss, impairment of ability to carry out multiple tasks (such as driving), loss of insight, reduced judgement, paranoia, heightened level of aggression, hallucinations (usually visual), confusion, disorientation and panic. Toxic reactions and psychosis associated with paranoia, hallucinations, bizarre or violent behaviour are well documented. Other physical symptoms include headache, nausea, inco-ordination, and dry mouth with physical signs including reduction in body temperature, red eyes, nystagmus, reduced blood pressure, tachycardia, increased respiratory rate.

Tolerance does develop, especially with prolonged use in high doses. Symptoms of withdrawal including anxiety, insomnia, headache, muscle cramps, sweating and mood disturbance may occur.

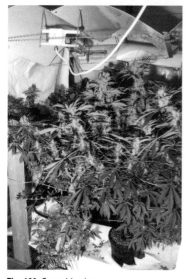

Fig. 160 Cannabis plant.

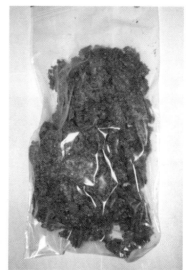

Fig. 161 Cannabis flower heads.

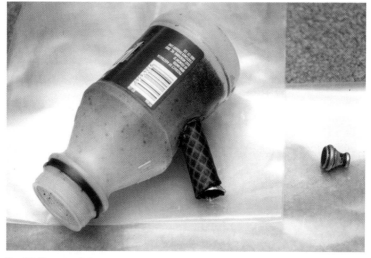

Fig. 162 Home made bong.

Stimulants are drugs that stimulate the central nervous system, peripheral nervous system and cardiovascular system. The group includes amphetamines (Fig. 163), cocaine, appetite suppressants such as phentermine, nicotine and caffeine.

The physical effects include reduced appetite with weight loss, nausea and vomiting, increased energy, tremor, restlessness, tachycardia with the risk of arrhythmia, dilated pupils and increase in body temperature. Psychological effects include euphoria, decreased fatigue and need for sleep, insomnia, anxiety, emotional lability and irritability and impairment of judgement. Paranoia and aggressive or violent outbursts, hallucinations, confusion or depression may also be apparent.

Tolerance to stimulant drugs develops within hours or days. Physical and psychological dependence also occurs, especially if high doses of the stimulant have been used. Withdrawal is manifested by muscle aches and pains, intense cravings for the drug, agitation, depression and insomnia.

After a few hours or days, there is an increase in appetite and somnolence. The persistent desire to use the drug associated with fatigue, anxiety, insomnia and depression may last for months or years. As with opiates, rehabilitation should be continued long term because of the likelihood of relapse.

Cocaine
Cocaine is sold on 'the streets' as an impure powder containing 1–20% cocaine, the remainder being inert substances such as glucose (Fig. 164).

Cocaine is absorbed well through all modes of administration but is usually 'snorted' intranasally or injected intravenously. 'Crack' or 'rock' cocaine is a crystallized form, which is smoked (Fig. 165). The effects of all types of cocaine are similar but 'crack' has a more rapid onset of action and more intense effects. After smoking or intravenous use, the peak blood levels are reached within 5–30 minutes but most of the drug disappears after 2 hours. Some activity may last for up to 4 hours. ➡

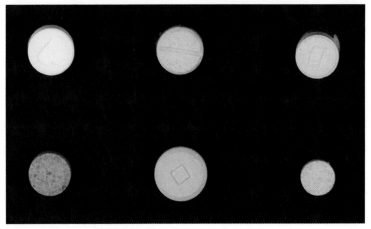

Fig. 163 Various tablet forms of amphetamines.

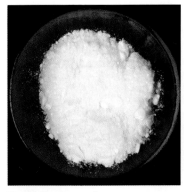

Fig. 164 Cocaine powder.

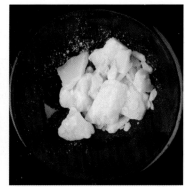

Fig. 165 'Crack' cocaine crystals.

Methylamphetamine

Methylamphetamine is sold on the streets as powder, crystal or gel. Crystal and gel may reach 60% purity, making it a very potent drug. It may be easily manufactured from easily obtainable precursors such as pseudoephedrine and ephedrine. It may be taken orally, intranasally or by intravenous injection. Large doses of up to 1 g methylamphetamine six to eight times a day can be tolerated by an experienced user. The drug is often used in a 'run', using the drug continuously for 2–4 days. This pattern of use is often associated with severe withdrawal ('crash') or psychosis.

Phentermine, fenfluramine, diethylpropion

These are drugs commonly prescribed to assist weight loss but they are also abused for their stimulant effects by truck drivers, students studying for exams and other individuals who want to remain awake for some reason. Abusers of these drugs may demonstrate paranoia, emotional lability or even aggressive or violent behaviour; this may lead to road-rage, associated accidents and dangerous driving incidents.

Hallucinogens

Hallucinogens include LSD (lysergic acid diethylamide) (Fig. 166), magic mushrooms (psylocybin), PCP (phencyclidine) and MDMA (ecstasy) (Fig. 167). These may produce a change in the level of consciousness and are capable of producing hallucinations.

Effects

All of these drugs are well absorbed when taken orally. Their potency varies with different side effect profiles. However, in lower doses most cause euphoria and increased self-awareness. Hallucinations (usually visual) occur in higher doses. The 'high' from LSD has a duration of hallucinations lasting from 8 to 12 hours. The 'high' experienced is dependent on the user's emotional state, prior drug experiences, psychiatric history and social environment.

Tolerance may develop within a few days. Dependence is unlikely and there is no withdrawal syndrome.

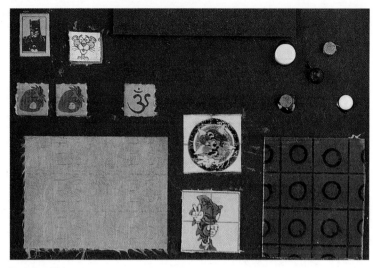

Fig. 166 LSD for sale.

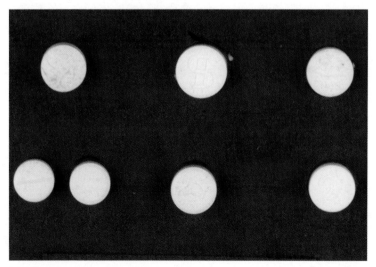

Fig. 167 Various tablet forms of ecstasy.

12 Specimen collection

Locard's principle (see page 3) is the fundamental guiding principle that underlies the approach to any crime scene examination. It states that whenever two objects come in contact with each other there is always transference of material from one to the other. Therefore, material from a victim may be found at the scene or on the offender, material from the offender may be found at the scene or on the victim, material from the scene may be found on the victim or offender.

Forensic specimens are specimens taken as evidence for the purpose of investigation of an offence. They may be taken from a crime scene or from a person. They enable the victim, perpetrator of the crime and the crime scene to be linked. Crime scene specimens are usually taken by a Scientific or Crime Scene Officer at the scene of a crime (Fig. 168). Taking of intimate and medical evidence specimens from a person is more likely to be the responsibility of a medical practitioner so it is important to understand the basic principles before a sample is taken. The correct sampling equipment must be used (Fig. 169) and samples handled appropriately so that the evidence obtained from those specimens is admissible in a court of law.

Consent

When any form of forensic specimen is taken from a person, written, informed consent of that person is required – whether or not the person is a complainant or a defendant in the investigation of an offence. Careful explanation must be given relating to the nature of the specimens being taken and the purpose for which they will be used. If a person is not competent to consent because of injury, intellectual or psychiatric disability or is a child, the consent is sought from a court of law, a court-appointed authorized person, a parent or next of kin. The type of consent and mechanisms for obtaining that consent will differ according to the jurisdiction in which the medical practitioner is working. ➡

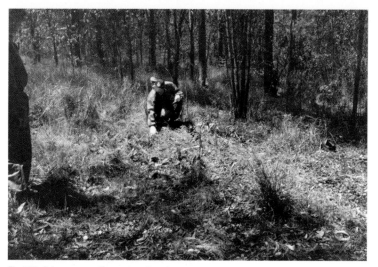

Fig. 168 Crime scene officers at a crime scene.

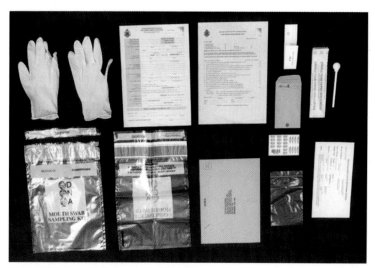

Fig. 169 DNA sampling kit – contents with tamper-proof bag.

Consent for taking samples from offenders or suspects is usually regulated by legislation. If appropriate consent is not sought, the results of any investigations may be deemed to be inadmissible in a court of law. The consent may be voluntary or an order may be made by a court for certain samples to be taken with or without the consent of the offender.

Types of sample

There are two types of specimens that may be taken from persons involved in offences.

- *Crime scene or medical evidence samples* are taken from a person and may link that person to another or to a scene implicated in the offence. Examples include vaginal swabs containing semen from a rape victim or spatters of blood swabbed from an offender after a murder.
- *Reference samples* are those with which the laboratory compares samples taken from the crime scene to identify a suspect or victim. The most common reference samples taken are buccal swabs or blood samples for DNA. Reference and medical evidence samples should always be kept separate to reduce the possibility of cross-contamination.

The containers used for specimens vary according to the laboratory but usually:

- blood sample placed in an EDTA tube for reference DNA (Fig. 170);
- buccal swab and FTA paper are used for reference DNA (Figs 171 and 172);
- unclotted blood placed in a potassium oxalate and sodium fluoride tube for alcohol and other drugs;
- urine placed in a sterile container for drug analysis;
- dry cotton wool swab sticks are used to swab for evidence;
- plastic clip seal bags are used for hairs, fibres, biological material such as leaves from clothing, foreign bodies from wounds, etc.;
- paper bags are used for dry clothing.

The types of samples taken from a victim will depend on the description of the assault by the victim and the findings on examination. ➡

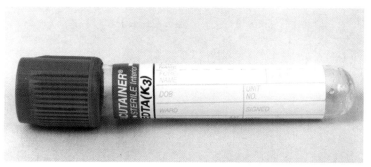

Fig. 170 EDTA specimen container for DNA analysis.

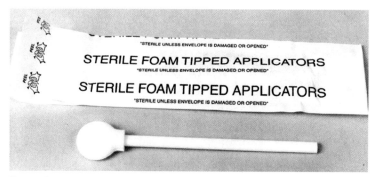

Fig. 171 Buccal swab for DNA collection.

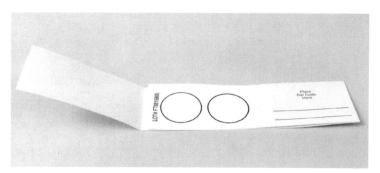

Fig. 172 FTA paper for DNA collection.

Table 2 illustrates typical forensic specimens taken from victims and suspects after a sexual assault.

Blood and urine specimens may also need to be taken for toxicology purposes in both criminal and traffic matters. Persons driving under the influence of alcohol or other drug may have to supply a blood sample within a certain period of time for the purpose of analysis for alcohol and other drugs. Unclotted blood is placed in a container with a preservative to prevent breakdown of the alcohol and some of the drugs. When taking a specimen of blood for blood alcohol a non-alcoholic swab should be used to clean the skin rather than one containing alcohol.

When drugs are suspected to have been used to facilitate a sexual assault or other crime, urine sampling is useful to perform a drug screen and may be positive for up to 4 days depending on the drug taken. A blood sample should be taken within 24 hours of the alleged assault.

Labelling and transportation

All specimens should be labelled with the following information:

- person's name;
- person's date of birth;
- doctor's name;
- date and time specimen taken;
- area sampled.

The samples should be sealed in tamper-proof bags or transport kits (see Fig. 169, p. 120). All biological samples should be dried before sealing and kept cold (but not frozen). Dry clothing should be placed in paper bags, wet clothing in plastic bags. The samples should be handed over to the investigating police officer or laboratory scientist. Whenever evidential samples are handed to another person, the information should be noted on a log sheet so that continuity of evidence is assured. Material should be transferred to the laboratory as soon as possible after sampling to minimize degradation of biological matter.

Table 2 Evidential value of specimens that may be taken after sexual assault

Specimen type	Equipment used	Evidential value
Specimens taken from victim		
Cervical os, high vaginal, low vaginal, vulval swabs	Dry swab and slide	Identification of spermatozoa and DNA from body fluids from assailant
Perianal, rectal swabs	Dry swab and slide	Identification of spermatozoa and DNA from body fluids from assailant
Swab of bite	Wet and dry swabs	Buccal cells for DNA analysis
Nail clippings, scrapings or swabs from nails	Nail clippers or scissors, orange stick or tooth picks	Blood or epithelial cells for DNA analysis from suspect if victim scratched suspect
Pubic combings	Comb and cotton wool	Stray hairs or fibres from the suspect
Blood or urine	Fluoride/oxalate or plain specimen container	Drugs used to facilitate sexual assault
Clothing	Paper bag	Semen, hair, fibres, blood from suspect or scene
Victim undresses on a drop sheet	Clean paper sheet	Biological matter, hairs and fibres may assist identification of suspect or scene
Blood or buccal swab	EDTA specimen container for blood or swab or FTA paper	Reference sample for DNA of victim
Specimens taken from suspect		
Swabs from base and shaft of penis	Dry swab	Vaginal or rectal mucosal cells from victim
Nail clippings, scrapings or swabs from nails	Nail clippers or scissors, orange stick or tooth picks	Vaginal or anal cells from victim if digital penetration suspected
Swab from bite	Wet and dry swabs	Saliva with buccal cells from the complainant for DNA analysis if victim bit the suspect
Blood	EDTA specimen container for blood or swab or FTA paper	Reference sample for DNA of suspect
Clothing	Paper bag	Blood, hair, fibres from victim or scene

13 Blood stains

In many jurisdictions, the documentation and analysis of blood stains is undertaken by scientists and police with doctors having a very limited, if any, input. Blood stains may, however, assist the doctor in interpreting events occurring at a scene including movement of the subject, and the direction and number of blows received. Blood stains are common at scenes where an injury has caused bleeding and will be on the victim and perhaps the surrounds. There are several points to consider when interpreting blood stains:

- Is it blood? (There are tests that will confirm this.)
- Damage to an artery causes blood spurts whereas venous damage causes blood to ooze out without any projection.
- When a sharp or blunt blow is delivered to a body causing an injury that bleeds (e.g. hammer blow to the scalp), there is a delay in that bleeding and it is usually at least the second blow to that site before the weapon will pick up blood and the motion cause blood splatter.
- Any motion of the bleeding site may cause blood splatter (Fig. 173).
- Direct contact of the bleeding site with a surface or object will cause blood markings, either as a direct marking or a smear (Fig. 174).
- Other persons (including the assailant) coming in contact with blood (including the bleeding site) may contribute to the disbursement of blood and cause both splatter and direct contact marks.
- When blood spots fly through the air and hit a surface, they leave a pattern which depends upon the angle and force of impact (e.g. a hit at right angles will result in a circular stain which will have spikes if forcible; oblique angle splashes will give a tapered stain with the sharp end pointing in the direction of travel) (Fig. 175).
- Blood oozing onto the victim's skin and clothing will track under gravity, dry and may provide information about the posture of the victim after wounding (Fig. 176).

Fig. 173 Blood splatter on a wall occurring during an assault.

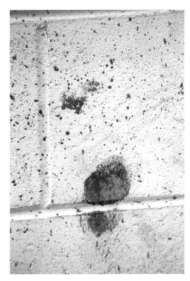

Fig. 174 Blood splatter and a blood smear from a victim with a head injury.

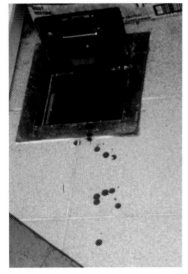

Fig. 175 Circular blood spots on the ground near an in-ground safe.

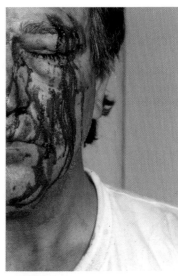

Fig. 176 Tracks of blood oozing from a laceration on the forehead.

14 Photography

Photography is an essential medicolegal tool. Well and appropriately taken photographs can supplement the clinical notes and positively contribute to the medicolegal case. On the other hand, poorly taken photographs and the interpretation of photographs without an understanding of their limitations can have disastrous outcomes in courts and tribunals. It should be remembered that any photograph taken of a patient for medical purposes becomes part of that patient's medical file.

Equipment

Suitable equipment can be expensive. An SLR camera with a macro lens (the lens should be of good quality) and flash light or equivalent digital camera system are preferred. When using a digital camera the quality and image size need to be high (preferably using tagged-image file format (TIFF); 1600×1200 pixels or higher) to allow suitable reproduction. A measuring and colour scale are essential items (Fig. 177). The colour scale is used to permit colour standardization and should be included in the first photo taken of each subject. Any scale used must not cover the injury being photographed (as it may be in Fig. 178). To avoid this, photos with and without the scale should be taken. A photograph should contain sufficient information to orient the viewer but should also highlight and provide suitable detail of the subject. Figure 179 shows the bruising on a child's leg but the nappy is more prominent and distracting. Photography of bruising is difficult. A bruise visible to the naked eye may not be evident on a photograph (Fig. 177). Similarly, some lesions and injuries not visible under certain lighting to the naked eye may be visible in a photograph taken with a flash light.

Labelling

Standard photographs should be labelled with the photographer's name, the subject's name, and the date and time the photograph was taken. Any digital images taken should be downloaded onto a CD for storage.

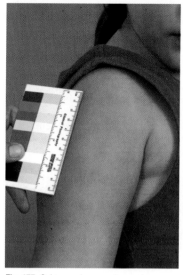

Fig. 177 Colour and measuring scale.

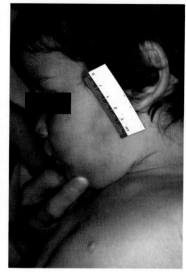

Fig. 178 Scale adjacent to or over bruise?

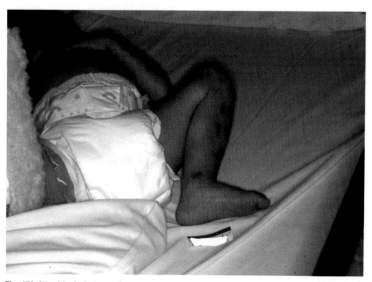

Fig. 179 Non-ideal photograph.

Index

abdominal bruising 26
abrasion collar 49
abrasions 29, 31, 32
  anal 95
  causes 31
  definition 31
  early healing 32
  with incisions 35
  sea lice damage 19
  self-inflicted 52
  in sexual assault 65, 67
    child abuse 91
  with stab wounds 37
abstinence syndrome 109
abusive head trauma 87
accidental death 5, 6
adipocere 11–13
  formation 12, 13
age and bruising 25
ageing
  abrasions 31
  bruises 29, 30
    in children 74
  incisions 35
  of injuries 23
alcohol 103–4
  absorption/metabolism 103
  and driving 123
  peak levels/elimination 103
amphetamines 117
  illicit laboratory 105–7
  tablet forms 116
amputations 55
anaemia and hypostasis 9
anal dilation 95, 96
anal examination 95
anal injuries, abuse-associated 95, 96
anal laxity/flaccidity 95
anaphylactoid purpura 77
animal predation 19, 20
appetite suppressants 117
autolysis, septic 17
autopsy 3
avulsion fractures 41

bags, paper/plastic 121
bags, plastic 121
'battered child syndrome' 81, 85
beating, scars from 55
benzodiazepines 111
  available preparations 112
bite marks 27, 74

human 39, 40
  adult vs immature 73
  vs animal 73
  in sexual assault 65, 67
  see also tooth marks
blanching 9
blisters 43
bloating 15, 16
blood alcohol levels 103
  sampling equipment 104, 123
blood loss and hypostasis 7
blood samples/sampling 123
  kit 104
  motor vehicle accidents 103
blood spots, shape of 125
blood stains 125–6
  interpretation 125
  types 126
body charts 23, 24
body fluid outflow see putrefactive ooze
body piercing 21, 50
bong, home-made 114
brain oedema 88
branding 55
bridging strands 33
  incisions vs lacerations 34
bruising 25–9
  ageing of 29, 30
  in child abuse 69, 71, 73
  from compression 60
  deep tissue 71
  definition 25
  delayed presentation 25
  factors affecting 25
  imprints 27
  patterns 27, 28, 56
  photography of 127, 128
  in sexual assault 65
  site 25
  skin colour 25, 29, 75
  with stab wounds 37
  vs hypostasis 11
  see also specific types of bruises
buccal swabs 121, 122
'bucket handle' fracture 83, 84
bullae 17, 18
bullous impetigo 83, 84
buprenorphine 109
burns 43, 58
  abuse-associated patterns 79–82
  conditions mistaken for 83
  multiple distinct 79, 80

outline   79
steam iron   80
symmetrical   81, 82
from torture   55
buscopan   109
buttocks, bruising of   75

cadaveric spasm   13–14
cannabis   113–14
Cannabis sativa   113, 114
carbon monoxide poisoning   11, 12
carpet burns   43, 44
chemical burns   43
child abuse
    crime scene   2
    cutaneous trauma   69–77
    fingertip bruising   27
    fractures   41
    physical   69–89
        objects used   71, 72
    sexual   89–96
        examination techniques   89, 90
        recognition   89
    cigarette burns   43, 67
        child abuse   79, 80
        impetigo mistaken for   83
classical metaphyseal lesion   83, 84
clinical forensic medicine   1
clonazepam   111
clonidine   109
close range projectile injuries   45, 46, 48
clothing
    and burns   43
    examination   59
    external examination   21
    in motor vehicle accidents   101
    of sexual assault victim   63
    spared in self-injury   51, 59, 60
coagulation disorders   77
cocaine   115, 116
codeine   107
cold rigor   13
colour of injuries   23
colour scale, photographic   127, 128
comminuted crush fractures   41
compression, petetchial bruises
following   27, 28
conditions mistaken for abuse   77
    burns   83
    fractures   85
    genital injuries   91, 97, 98
consent
    to forensic examination   61
    to specimen collection   119, 121
contact burns   43, 44, 79
    accidental   79
contact projectile injuries   45–8
contusions *see* bruising
'corner chip' fracture   83, 84
corporal punishment   95

'crack' cocaine   115, 116
crime investigation protocols   3
crime scene   3–4, 120
    child abuse   2
    inspection of   51
    potential   2, 3
    specimens   119, 121
Crime Scene Officers   119, 120
cross-tolerance   111
crush fractures, comminuted   41
crush injuries   73
'cry for help' self injury   49

death
    categories   5–7
    scene of
        as potential crime scene   3
        securing   7
        preservation   7–8
        evidence from   7
    suspicious   3, 4
decomposition   9, 15
    tattoos, persistence during   21
defensive injuries   37, 53, 54
    absence of   53
    locations   53
    types   53
'degloved' appearance   17
delayed care seeking   81
dentists, forensic   39
dependence, drug   105
    benzodiazepines   111
    hallucinogens   118
    heroin   107, 109
    stimulants   115
dermatological conditions   77–8
diaphyseal fractures   85
diastasis ani   97
diazepam   109, 111
diethylpropion   117
digital cameras   127
direction of applied force   31
discoloration *see* skin colour
diseases and bruising   25
DNA evidence from bites   39
DNA sampling kit   120
documentation   51
    blood stains   125
    drawings of injuries   23
    photography   127
    potential torture victims   54
    recording external features   21
    recording injuries   23–4
    recording scene of death   7
    in sexual assault   63
    specimen collection   123
    weapon features   57
drowning, death by
    insect damage   19, 20

maceration 17
marbling 18
drug abuse
    evidence of 21, 22
    see also drugs, illicit
drug screens 123
drugs
    and alcohol 103
    and bruising 25
    illicit 105–18
        effects 105
        package examples 108
        treatment programmes 107
        types 107
    physical effects
        benzodiazepines 111
        cannabis 113
        heroin 107
        stimulants 115
    psychological effects
        benzodiazepines 111
        cannabis 113
        heroin 107
        stimulants 115
    use/abuse 105
duodenal damage 87

ear piercing 50
ears
    damage 63
    petetchial bruises 75, 76
ecstasy 117, 118
EDTA tubes 121, 122
electrical burns 43, 44
    from torture 55
entry wounds
    rifled weapons 45
    smooth bore weapons 47
entomologists, forensic 19
environmental conditions
    and decomposition 9
    and putrefaction 15
    scene of death 7
equipment 1
    blood alcohol sampling 104, 123
    DNA sampling 120
    forensic/doctor's bag 2
    photography 2, 127
    sampling 119
erythema 29, 91
ethanol 103
ethnic origin 21, 22
evidence
    DNA, from bites 39
    drug abuse 21, 22
    kit 62
    of medical conditions 21, 22
    medical, specimens of 119, 121
    from scene of death 7

examination *see also specific types of*
    examination
    of clothing 51, 59
    consent to 61
    external features 9, 21–2
    of sexual assault victim
        child 89, 90
        external 63
    weapons 57
exit wounds
    rifled weapons 45
    smooth bore weapons 47, 48
external examination 9, 57
    of clothing 59
    sexual assault victim 63

facial bruising
    with immune thrombocytopenic
        purpura 78
    in young children 75
facial injuries 63, 64
facial swelling 15, 16
failure of midline fusion 97, 98
fenfluramine 117
fingernail abrasions 31, 32, 73
fingernail/toenail damage 55
fingertip bruising 28, 31
    child abuse 69
    in sexual assault 27, 65, 67
fire
    death by 15, 16
    injuries from 43
fissures, perianal 95
flunitrazepam 111
fly infestation 19, 20
foreign material
    incisions *vs* lacerations 34
    in motor vehicle accidents 101
    speculum examination for 63
    in wounds 33
forensic dentists 39
forensic entomologists 19
forensic evidence kit 62
forensic medicine 1
forensic physicians 1, 3
forensic specimens 67
    belonging to attacker 67
fractures 41, 42
    abuse, mistaken for 85
    abuse-associated 83, 84–5
    dating of 85
    direct/indirect force 41
    in motor vehicle accidents 101
friction burns 43, 44
FTA paper 121, 122

gas 15
gas formation 15
genital examination 65, 89, 90
genital injuries

abuse, mistaken for   97–8
abuse-associated
    female acute   91, 92
    female healed   93, 94
    accidental   93, 97
    conditions mistaken for   91
    male   95
genital structures   90
gingival damage   63, 64
granulation tissue   31, 91, 92
greenstick fractures   41
grip marks/bruising   27, 28, 69, 70

haematomas
    abdominal   90
    genital   91
    penile   96
    scrotal   88, 96
haemophilias   77
hair in mummification   19
half-life, THC   113
hallucinogens   117–18
hand marks   68, 69
handcuffs   57
head injury   87
healing
    recording of   23
    time taken   91
heat rigor   13
Henoch Schoenlein purpura   77
heroin   107, 109, 110
'high tide line'   81, 82
history, inconsistent   69, 79, 87
history-taking
    motor vehicle accidents   101
    potential self-injury   51
    potential torture victims   55
    sexual assault, adult   61, 63
'hit and run' cases   101
homicide   5, 6
humerus, fractures of   86
hymen
    adolescent   93, 94
    clefts/notches/concavities   91, 94
    damage to   91, 92
        accidental   97
    examination of   89
    neonatal   93
    transection   93, 94
hymenal narrowing   93, 94
hyper/hypopigmentation   71
hypostasis   9–11
    blanching/fixing   9, 10
    and skin slippage   17
    sparing in pressure areas   9–11
    vs bruising   9
    vs carbon monoxide poisoning   11

ibuprofen   108
illicit drugs see drugs, illicit

impetigo   83, 84
imprints   27
incisions   35–6
    causes   35
    defensive injuries   54
    self-inflicted   50, 52
    vs lacerations   33, 34
incomplete fractures see greenstick
    fractures
infant deaths, hidden   19
injuries   23–60
    abuse, mistaken for   77, 78
    abuse-associated   77
    actual vs expected   59, 69
    description/recording   23–4
    features recorded   23
    from forcible restraint   67
    interpretation   67
    shape of   23
    size of   23
    from torture   67
insect infestation   19, 20
interchange, Locard's theory of   3, 119
internal injuries
    abuse-associated   87, 88
    torture-associated   54
intravaginal ridges   97
intravenous drug abuse   105, 106
    paraphenalia   108
    and staphylococcal sepsis   110
    treatment, relapse from   111
intravenous marks/track sites   106
in-utero degeneration   17
ischaemia, penile   95
isotopic bone scans   41

jejunal damage   87
jewellery   21

keratin nodules   43
'knee chest' position   89, 90

labial traction   89, 90
lacerations   33
    anal   95, 96
    causes   33
    genital   91, 92
    locations   33
    from torture   54
    vs incisions   33, 34
laxity of tissue   25
legal issues see medicolegal issues
lichen sclerosis et atrophicus   97, 98
ligation, penile   95
ligature marks   55, 56
    in child abuse   73, 74
linea vestibularis   97, 98
liquefaction   17
liver, damage to   89
livor mortis (lividity) see hypostasis

Locard's theory of interchange 3, 119
lofexidine 109
Lomotril 109
long bones, fractures of 83
long range projectile injuries 45, 47
'love bites' 27, 39, 40
    penile 95
    in sexual assault 65
LSD (lysergic acid diethylamide)
   117–18

maceration 17, 18
magic mushrooms 117
malingering 49
manslaughter 5
marbling 15, 17, 18
margins of injuries 23
    incisions 35
    incisions vs lacerations 34
marijuana see cannabis
MDMA 117
measuring scale, photographic 127,
   128
medical conditions
    associated with drug use 105–7
    evidence of 21, 22
medical evidence specimens 119, 121
medicolegal issues
    injuries, description/recording of 23
    motor vehicle accidents 101
    photography 127
    specimen collection 119
    suicide 99
metaclopramide 109
metaphyseal damage 85
metaphyseal lesion, classical 83, 84
methadone 107
methylamphetamine 117
migration of bruises 25
'mirror image' burns 81, 82
misadventure 5
moisture and adipocere formation 11
mongolian spots 77, 78
morphine 107
motor vehicle accidents 101–2
    alcohol and 103
    injuries 101
motor vehicle occupants 101
mouth, examination of 63
movement of body and hypostasis 11
multidisciplinary support team 3
mummification 19–20
Munchausen's syndrome 49

naevus, congenital, simulating black eye
   78
narcotic analgesics 107, 109–11
natural death 5, 6, 7
neck injuries 63, 64
    defensive 53

nitrazepam 111
nomenclature of injuries 23

oblique fracture 41
odour of adipocere 11
oedema 29, 30
    abrasion-associated 31
    brain 88
    child sexual abuse 91
    after penile ligation 95
opiates 107
ornaments 21
osteogenesis imperfecta 85, 86

paddling bruises 75
pancreas, damage to 87
paracetamol 109
patterned injuries 59
    child abuse 69–73
    skeletal injury 83
    von Willebrand's disease 76, 77
patterned scars 55
PCP 117
pedestrians 101
periorbital bruising 26
    following forehead/scalp injury 25
petetchial bruises 27, 28, 63
    child abuse 69, 71
    child sexual abuse 89
    ears 75, 76
    locations 39
    penile 95, 96
pH and adipocere 11
pharyngeal laceration 87
phencyclidine 117
phentermine 117
photography 51, 127–8
    equipment 2, 127
    labelling 127
    pitfalls 127, 128
    recording injuries 23
physeal cartilage, damage to 83
physical abuse, child see under child
   abuse
physical dependence, drug 105
pigmentary lesions 77
pinch marks 73, 74
pneumoperitoneum 90
poly-drug use 111
port wine stain 78
positioning for genital examination 63,
   89, 90
post-mortem changes 9–20
post-mortem sparing 9
potassium oxalate/sodium fluoride tube
   121
powder burns 45
powder tattooing 45
predation 19
preservation of features

with adipocere   11
in mummification   19
proctoscope examination   65
projectile injuries
 high velocity   45
 low velocity   45
 rifled weapons   45
 smooth bore weapons   45
promethazine   109
pruritis   97
psychiatric disorders   49, 50
psychological conditions   105–7
psychological dependence, drug   105
psylocybin   117
'pugilistic position'   13, 14
putrefaction   15–18
 conditions affecting   15
 putrefactive changes   8, 18
putrefactive ooze   15, 16

radiation burns   43
radiography   83
'railway line' bruising   27
rape kit   62
'read-back' alcohol graphs   103, 104
recording see documentation
reference samples   121
retinal haemorrhages   87, 88
rib fractures   83, 84
rigor mortis   13, 14
 delayed by cold rigor   13
'rock' cocaine   115, 116

sample handling   119
sampling equipment   2, 119
 DNA   120
saponification   11
scalds   43
 child abuse   81–2
scarring, anal   95
sea lice damage   19, 20
self-injury   49, 50
 abrasions/incisions   52, 58, 60, 67
 bruising   67
 consequences of diagnosis   51
 features of   51
 incisions   35, 36
 for secondary gain   49
 and sexual assault   67
 sparing of clothing   59, 60
 types   49
semen detection   63
sepsis, staphylococcal   110
septic autolysis   17
serosanguinous fluid   16
sexual abuse, child see under child
 abuse
sexual assault
 adult   61–8
 forensic examination   61, 62, 63, 65

frequency of injuries   67
 male victims   65
 response   61
bite marks in   39
child see child abuse, sexual
fingertip bruising   27
specimen collection   124
'shaken baby' syndrome   87, 88
shotgun wounds   45, 47, 48
skeletal injury   83–7
 abuse-associated   83, 85, 86
 see also fractures
skeletonization   15
skin colour
 bruising   25, 27, 29, 75
 carbon monoxide poisoning   11,
  12
 hypostasis   9, 11
 putrefaction   15–18
 putrefactive changes   15
skin pigmentation and bruising   25
skin slippage/lift   15, 17, 18
 fly larvae in   20
skin tags   31, 32
slap marks   69, 70
slashes see incisions
slate-grey spots   77, 78
specialist expertise   7
specimen collection   119–24
 after sexual assault   123
 equipment   2, 119, 120
 labelling/transportation   123
 from suspect   124
 from victim   124
specimen containers   121
specimen types   121
specimens, evidential value   124
speculum examination   63
spiral fracture   41, 42
stab wounds   37
 appearance   37, 38
 causes   37
 classification   37
 suicidal   37, 38, 50
stimulants   115–18
strangulation, fingertip bruising in   27
subarachnoid haematoma   87
subconjunctival haemorrhage   39, 40,
 63, 64
subdural haematoma   87, 88
submucosal haemorrhage   91, 92
substance use/misuse   105
suction bruises   65
 penile   95
 see also 'love bites'
suicide   5, 99–100
 methods   99
 suspected   7
swab sticks   121
swabs of sexual assault victim   65

tattoos 21, 22
temazepam 111
tenderness 29
Δ-9-tetrahydrocannabinol (THC) 113
thigh injuries, defensive 53
thrombocytopenic purpura,
  idiopathic/immune 77, 78
timing
    hypostasis 9
    putrefaction 15
    rigor mortis 13
timing of injuries *see under* ageing
tissue binding of THC 113
tolerance to drugs 105
    benzodiazepines 111
    cannabis 113
    hallucinogens 117
    heroin 107
    stimulants 115
tongue swelling/protrusion 16
tooth marks 95
   see also bite marks
torture 55, 56
'tramline' bruising 27, 28, 56
transport kits 123
transverse fracture 41, 86
tub immersion burn 81, 82

undetermined cause of death 7
upper limb injuries, defensive 53, 54
urethral prolapse 97, 98
urine samples 123

vaginitis 97
vascular lesions 77
vehicular damage 101, 102
von Willebrand's disease 76, 77

'washerwoman's hands' 17, 18
weapons 58
    documentation of features 57
    examination 57
    handling/contamination 57
whipping, scars from 55
withdrawal, drug 105
    benzodiazepines 111
    heroin 109
    methadone 109
    methylamphetamine 117
    stimulants 115
    symptomatic treatment 109
    symptoms/signs 109
wounds
    contents of 23
    foreign material in 33